Much More to Come

Much More to Come

Lessons on the mayhem and
magnificence of midlife

Eleanor Mills

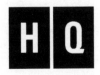

ONE PLACE. MANY STORIES

HQ
An imprint of HarperCollins*Publishers* Ltd
1 London Bridge Street
London SE1 9GF

www.harpercollins.co.uk

HarperCollins*Publishers*
Macken House, 39/40 Mayor Street Upper
Dublin 1, D01 C9W8, Ireland

This edition 2024

1
First published in Great Britain by
HQ, an imprint of HarperCollins*Publishers* Ltd 2024

A catalogue record for this book is
available from the British Library.

HB ISBN: 978-0-00-864256-3

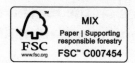

To Derek, Alice and Laura with love and gratitude

CONTENTS

INTRODUCTION

By the time we reach fifty, over half of women have been through at least five big life challenges, including: divorce, bereavement, redundancy, abuse, bankruptcy, illness, coping with tricky teenagers, or elderly parents falling ill and dying. Not to mention our own health issues and menopause. Often, these challenges hit us all at once in a midlife maelstrom, leaving us spluttering and stranded. And because we are a pioneering generation of women – one of the first to reap the benefits of greater equality – there is no guide for how to pick ourselves up and persevere; no map for what our lives could look like from here on.

This book provides that map, drawing on inspiring tales of how women have survived and thrived; how they moved into, through and beyond adversity in midlife. This is a positive book – a guide for how women can make the most of their third quarter. It's a rallying cry for a new kind of woman hitting midlife. For, after all, if many of us will live to nearly 100 years old, fifty is only halfway through. The old map may have run out but there is so much more life still to come. And midlife women have the wisdom and strength to see these years through – they just need to know what the next phase might look like.

I hit my own midlife maelstrom when I was made redundant from the job that had defined me for twenty-five years. I searched in vain for a guide to what came next, for what the next version of me might look like and what I needed to do to find it. The redundancy section of the

HMRC website was *not* what I needed. Nor was scrolling through lists of 'Things To Do When You've Been Fired'. I couldn't find anything out there to help me navigate my next chapter.

So, for the last number of years, I have been on a journey of discovery. I have pulled myself back up again after a professional whacking, through a mixture of hard work, determination, bloody-mindedness and rage that the world was writing off women like me when we still had so much to offer. I knew from a decade of being a weekly newspaper columnist on the UK's highest-selling broadsheet that if I was exercised about something then other people probably were too – so I set up Noon, a community for women pivoting in midlife, and started gathering stories to inspire other women not to give up. I've always loved the phrase, 'You can't be what you can't see.' I wanted other women who felt lost and on the scrap heap in midlife to look at Noon and read my story and know that they weren't done, it wasn't over, there was a path to reinvention and a good act to follow. That there is a positive answer to that dreaded question: what next?

I like to think of fifty as the age when we finally become the women we always wanted to be. It's why I coined the term Queenagers. I wanted to communicate that sense of us coming into our prime, becoming our true selves – a kind of through-the-pupa-and-out-of-the-chrysalis period when we spread our wings into our own brave new worlds like midlife butterflies. The word Queenager was inspired in part by a woman in one of our Noon focus groups who said, 'I feel like a teenager, but in my own house, with good sheets and proper tea.' I was also inspired by my frequent trips to Jamaica, where they talk about women as 'queens', which I love. In my funny old headline-writing brain the two ideas came together and – boom! – Queenager was born. I'm proud to say it was listed in roundups of 2022 as one of the new words of the year and is catching on fast, having made appearances all over the UK press and now the *Washington Post* and Bloomberg too. For me, it sums up the experience and transitional nature of this time in a woman's life:

that we are in a kind of young-old phase – a bit hormonal, in a period of change but packing wisdom and dignity – midlife queens, if you like. Queenagers.

I love stories. As a journalist, ink is in my blood. So this book is full of the conversations that have helped shape my transition into a new, happier, more whole version of myself; accounts gleaned from the community of women in midlife that I have created at Noon and through my bestselling Substack newsletter, *The Queenager* (one of the ten most read globally last year). My audience responds to the optimism of the tales I tell about this transition; these stories of transformation that become the stepping stones to our own reinventions. These tales are like the white pebbles which shone in the moonlight for Hansel and Gretel and provided a path out of the dark wood, away from the wicked witch's house and safely home. *Much More to Come* is the guide I was seeking when I was lost in that midlife wood. I hope it helps point the way for others.

In fact, I want all the women following along after me to look forward to being fifty as the point when they come into their prime as Queenagers – not dread it. Women have no sell-by date! Women of fifty today are pioneers – we are feeling our way to a new kind of later-life adventure. While on this journey, I have created a new vocabulary to help us talk about this time in our lives, which you can find in the glossary at the end of this book.

Of course every loss leaves a hole, but what I've learnt is that in that void something wonderful can grow – if we have the support and confidence to let it. At fifty, we women aren't done, unseen, invisible, all the things popular culture would have us believe. We are just getting going. Just hitting our stride. As one Queenager put it to me: 'I feel like I am just getting the hang of things.' But we need to hear these stories in order to emulate them. We need to see what others have done in order to recreate and reimagine what the later stages of women's lives can look like.

You can read this book from the beginning, or you can dip in and out, to focus on a story that relates to something specific you are going through today. The sections are there as signposts to help you through your own dark time into a brighter future. This book is a bit like a patchwork quilt – the stories hang together as a narrative or can be dipped into individually. The story of my own becoming weaves them together. At forty-nine I thought my life was going swimmingly – then the bottom fell out of my world and I had to reinvent it from scratch. And I am not the only one. Many of us have spent the first two twenty-five-year chunks of our lives playing out other people's expectations, looking after others, putting our own dreams aside. Well, the good news is that fifty – when we hit the third quarter of our lives – is *our* time, when it finally is all about us. And no, it's not too late, and you aren't too old!

What all these stories from women all over the world, in midlife, moving through trying times into better ones demonstrate is that in the darkest moments there is always light, just as the black of a shadow can accentuate the brightness of the most sparkling day. When I was a young woman, I loved Erica Jong's *Fear of Flying* – it summed up how women felt as they set out from the shores of the sexual revolution, relishing the freedom but also trepidatious about the unknown. *Much More to Come* is a similar positive, poignant guide.

It is time for a new script. I offer these tales from midlife to encourage you on your journey, wherever you are. I found that these conversations buoyed me up when times were tough. I hope these women who share their stories can inspire you just as they did me. I also offer you my own story. I know that it is a tale of privilege – I admit I am a white, privately educated Cis woman, born in London, which is an extraordinarily lucky bit of inheritance – but there is so little out there tackling the midlife maelstrom for women that I hope I have something to offer this discussion. This book is intended to lift you up when you are down, and light the way to the next part of your life.

Maybe it will help you through a bad day or provide suggestions to guide you through the pinch points and on to the sunny uplands of this stage in life: not caring what others think and instead living and speaking your own truth. Researching and sharing these stories guided me on to a new and happier phase in my life. I hope that with the help of this book and all these wise women you will find your way there too. It is okay to find it difficult. It *is* difficult. But if we dare to dream, we can do it – and our individual stories of flourishing and living well from midlife onwards can build a whole new sense of what this time in life can look like. A whole new movement. I call it the Queenager Revolution. Come and join us!

Eleanor Mills
Noon.org.uk
April 2024

PART ONE

THE MIDLIFE MAELSTROM

My new life began on a bench. An ordinary wooden bench in the scruffy inner-city park behind my house. It's the kind of place where teens hang out and smoke marijuana. Where knackered parents push toddlers on rusting swings and dogs sniff each other while their owners fumble with scented plastic bags. It smells of pee and pavement. At dusk the graffitied metal gate is padlocked.

To this paradise, then, I went on a hot summer's day in lockdown to meet an old friend. She lives round the corner but we hadn't seen each other in a while – partly because of the pandemic but really because I'd been dodging her texts, sending her calls to voicemail. I'd just been made redundant and I couldn't face anyone. I was too sad. Too ashamed. Humiliated. Lost. It sounds mad now but in the aftermath of being let go, I felt like I had died. There was the same finality.

There was no way back to what had been my life. It was over. Gone. It happened with dizzying speed.

One moment all was normal. I'd come back from lunch, waved cheerily to my team and headed up to a meeting with the top boss, full of plans for the next few months. Then I was out. Whacked.

As legal papers were passed to and fro across the table it all felt far away. My mind had checked out. The conversation continued but I was swooping and diving with the pigeons on the roof of the church opposite. Watching a tug make slow progress against the frothing current on the river below. I couldn't take anything in. I just remember chanting to myself: 'Don't cry, don't cry, don't give them that satisfaction.' I'm proud to say that I didn't crack then. But nothing made sense.

My world stopped in that moment. In the ensuing months, my mind kept returning to those minutes in the boss's office like a moth to a flame. I'd be lying in bed and find myself back there, my heart racing. I was unable to process what had happened. How everything that had been familiar was over. That it was all gone. Afterwards I was in freefall, disorientated. I couldn't stop crying. The only place that felt safe was home; in bed, binge-watching *The Crown*. But that day my friend insisted ... and I hadn't the strength to resist.

When I got to the park, red eyes hidden by big gold sunglasses, she was already on the bench. Next to her was a Tesco carrier bag.

'Look! Pimm's!' She cracked open a tin and offered me one too. I took a long, warm, sugary swig. It was noon, on a Monday. It felt like rock bottom.

'How are you? I haven't seen you since ...' She trailed off. No one wanted to say the word. It *was* a bit like a death.

I tried to be cheerful. It is my trademark. But the upbeat words just wouldn't come. I'd spent thirty years telling stories, finding sexy angles – but I couldn't put a good gloss on this. There was a long pause. And then a big sob erupted from deep inside. My whole body shook. Despite social distancing, she edged closer and gave me a forbidden hug.

It all came tumbling out. Who was I without the job I'd spent half my life doing? Without that cloak of power, the status it lent me, what was I? It was like Darth Vader taking off the mask. I'd put the job ahead of so much, sometimes even my kids and my family. When the boss said 'Jump!' I leapt with alacrity. I'd worn the *Game of Thrones* power cloak for over two decades, while I had grown from a young gun to a middle-aged woman; it was part of me and now it was gone. I felt lost. A failure. A big tear plopped onto the bench. I took another swig of Pimm's. It was flat and the alcohol burnt my stomach. I took another, larger one.

I cried some more. I felt awful. On top of losing my job I'd had Covid and was physically weak and frail. I was staring down the barrel of my fiftieth birthday and felt every one of those long years. My eldest daughter was about to go to uni, leaving a yawning hole in my home. I was worried about money (I'd always been the main breadwinner and, now that I didn't have a job, I was racked with anxiety about what came next for all of us).

Even worse, all the inner doubts and gremlins – many from my childhood – which had been silenced by busyness, by worldly success, were now raising their painful heads. During that time my brain felt full of whirling knives, each thought worse than the one it replaced.

I felt like I was unravelling – in bright sunlight, on a bench with my friend, glugging a tin of tepid Pimm's.

I hiccupped and coughed, snotting my way through a pile of tissues. And do you know the best thing about that day? My friend didn't say: 'You'll bounce back!' or 'It'll all be fine!', like everyone else had. Quietly, she was just there, passing me tissues, patting my arm. Letting me feel my loss and my pain. There are times when we don't want to be fixed, we just want to be witnessed. To be held. To be heard.

'We can't go over it. We can't go under it. Oh, no! We've got to go through it.'

Like the children in Michael Rosen's *We're Going on a Bear Hunt*, who must swim across a river, splosh through mud and swish through long grass, there is no shortcut through the grief that accompanies the end of one life phase and the beginning of another. Just endurance. Sympathy helps, and distraction (TV, chocolate, Pimm's, hugs). But time is the real medicine. Time and being kind to ourselves.

Did you know that the necessity for a pause, for a wait in the darkness before life starts again, is the oldest story of them all? I didn't until a new friend sent me a book about an Assyrian goddess called Inanna. She was the Queen of Heaven and Earth and is the hero of one of humanity's earliest myths found etched on tablets of stone at the beginning of writing.

So, Inanna. Her sister Ereshkigal, Queen of the Underworld, is mourning the death of her husband. Inanna descends from her earthly kingdom down into the realm of the dead to attend the funeral rites. At each of the gates that guard the way to the underworld Inanna is forced to shed some of her mortal finery; first her golden ring, then her lapis beads – even her royal robe is taken. It is the beginning of a nightmare. Stripped naked, totally vulnerable, Inanna is imprisoned in the underworld by her grieving sister, and is unable to return to the light and the air.

> Then Ereshkigal fastened on Inanna the eye of death.
> She spoke against her the word of wrath.
> She uttered against her the cry of guilt.
> She struck her. Inanna was turned into a corpse.
> A piece of rotting meat.
> And was hung from a hook on a wall.

The goddess hangs there in the dark. Stuck, unable to move, lifeless. A hunk of decaying meat.

But in what looks like death, something surprising happens. Inanna is not dead, but fallow. Waiting. Like the earth in winter, she seems forgotten but she is actually regenerating, rebooting, renewing herself quietly, in the dark and the silence. Eventually, she is rescued by her mortal friends who come to look for her. She emerges from this time in the darkness way more powerful; wiser, brighter. She has regenerated and brought the spring, the renewal. Through her ordeal of being hung on the hook, she has managed to unite the worlds of the living and the dead. And she now rules as Queen in both.

So it is for us Queenagers. In midlife, we will go through dark times. Be hung on our own hooks. We probably won't be struck down by Ereshkigal, but the vast majority of us will get whacked by something. I have seen it over and over again – in our Noon Circles and in our research. What is for sure is that whatever has propelled us through the last twenty-five years of our life will end at around fifty. Whether it's the termination of a career, or a marriage, having to face illness – our own, or that of a child or parent – or bereavement or an empty nest, whatever shape our own midlife maelstrom (or midlife clusterfuck) takes, it often all hits at once and manifests as a kind of death that blows away everything we have known. In that moment many of us feel like it is all over. That what we were has died. That it is the end.

If that sounds familiar, please don't despair.

What I have learnt from my own experience and seen in all the thousands of midlife women who I've talked to is that, like Inanna, if we wait, if we are kind to ourselves and allow ourselves to sit in the dark and reflect and regenerate, and particularly when we engage the loving encouragement of family, friends and a supportive new community to help us into this next phase, then we – like the ancient Queen – can flourish again.

It's not easy. At the beginning, the path is steepest. The way ahead is unclear. Anxiety stalks us. Tears are legion. Our minds keep coming back to the loss, the pain, like worrying the hole in your mouth after a tooth extraction. It's horrible. It's painful. And inescapable.

I remember taking myself to a qigong class (like tai chi but easier) and at the end of the two-hour workshop (yup, not something I'd ever really done before, but hell, I had time on my hands ...) the instructor asked us all to say how we felt. He went around the class. The woman next to me said mystically she could feel energy charged between her hands crackling like rainbows (yeah, right). A bloke quoted something wise from a Chinese text. I was so choked up I couldn't speak. I also didn't have a hanky so was covered in teary snot. I mumbled something about having had some bad news and finding the transition tricky.

The teacher nodded and said, matter-of-factly, 'Change is difficult' before walking back to the front of the room. I am sure he had no idea what he had done. But all I can say is that his words were a tonic. He was the first person who had acknowledged where I was. That I was finding the change unbearably tough. That it was difficult. That I was a snotty, snivelling mess. Not coping at all. He was the first person who gave me permission to not be okay. Who acknowledged I was in a real hole and finding it tough. His recognition of where I found myself, his casual acceptance of it as fact, was a sweet relief. It was like hitting the bottom of a swimming pool and feeling concrete beneath my feet so that I could push back up.

Change is difficult. With those words I stopped feeling ashamed and furious about how pathetic and weak I was being, and for the first time I felt a little sympathy for myself. I accepted where I was: in a state. That I wasn't a failure for finding it tough. It *was* tough. And humiliating and worrying and disorientating. The shift was being told it was okay – even normal and acceptable – to find it so.

So that is what I hope these words will do for you too. Repeat them to yourself: *Change is difficult.* Pat yourself on the back that you are getting through it. Allow yourself to feel all of it. Sob on your friends, partner, family or children (mine got so used to me being teary that they'd joke about 'what the mum weather was like' that morning: drizzle, hard rain, deluge …). Remember, there are no quick fixes; that, like the first time you had your heart broken, only time can make it better. And that this phase will pass.

Give yourself a ticket to wallow. Lie around and watch sad films or binge-watch your favourites. Eat ice cream. Consider yourself hugged. Don't try to do anything. Shedding old identities and ways of being is hard. Particularly if you are used to being super-busy – I felt like one of those Indian deities with sixteen arms and nothing to do with any of them. Sit with it. Think of Inanna the Queen hanging on her hook, waiting in the dark, feeling it all. Locked in the underworld. Know that this is the only way; and remember that this is how that earliest of myths ends:

'You mount the steps to your high throne/ In all majesty you sit there/ Queenship and godship in your hands.'

It just sums it up. We can rise again, have a fantastic next chapter, move into the light and rediscover our joy. That is what the stories in this part of the book are all about. Inspiration that this too shall pass.

But first. Pause.

Please.

Change is difficult

This book is about becoming – becoming the women we always wanted to be, in midlife. It isn't all joyful. All change involves loss, a clearing out of what was, in favour of what could be. That sounds poetic but the reality is not. We are moving from something concrete, something that we have held in our hands, to a massive maybe … a future of question marks and uncertainty. Sure, it could be great. But it could get worse.

In my own journey of becoming, one of my lowest times was shortly after I was made redundant. It was March 2020, and I felt like I was in freefall: I would cry several times a day, and even worse than that was the anxiety – a constant gnawing in my stomach, a niggling in my mind. I would go for a walk and be flooded with fear and adrenaline about trivial things; whether the car would get a ticket, if I'd left the oven on at home. But also about practical matters such as how I would pay the mortgage. I'd picture unpaid bills, or worry about how I'd pay for my children to go to university. These practical fears lived alongside a more existential one about being done, washed up, finished. Fifty. My best days behind me.

Panic lurked in my gut. It could be kept at bay in the presence of others, or with constant distraction, but as soon as I was alone, or still, it became overwhelming. I was all at sea. I really felt redundant in the sense of having nothing to do. In my former job, I had felt intensely needed; at any given time there would be a queue of people wanting my attention, my decision, a response to their e-mail, a meeting. Now when I picked up my phone it was weirdly void. No one needed me anymore. It was like I no longer existed.

I'd always been warned that the graveyards were full of irreplaceable editors and CEOs, politicians and celebrities; that no job ever loves you back, that the only people to whom we are truly irreplaceable are our families. It is true. After decades of loyal service here I was: junked. Rejected. Thrown out like the rubbish. Cast out of my world, and my work tribe. The truth is that I just didn't know how to *be* if I was no longer that person. I know now that intense busyness was my go-to place. It was an addiction – a permanent distraction from feeling my feelings. Evicted from the job, made redundant, I was in a state of withdrawal, suffering like any addict craving a fix. And the fix was a feeling of being needed, being essential, feeling important. The endless dopamine hit of my phone pinging with things that needed my attention.

My best friend tried to help; she was about to go to Jamaica for ten days with a new beau and kindly invited me to go along as a third wheel. She thought a change of scene might do me good. But even watching waves crashing on the reef or the pelicans dive-bombing into the sea – two of my very favourite things – didn't help. I still couldn't relax or sleep. I paced around the small apartment where I was staying on my own and wondered why I had forsaken the solidity of home, my husband, my girls, to be alone thousands of miles away.

I remember lying in a hammock on a Jamaican mate's porch. The hammock was multicoloured and cheerful. His wide-eyed children were cute and playing around me in the garden. But I was stiff as a plank, rigid with tension, so full of fear that I was convinced the strings of the hammock would snap, unable to trust that it could keep me suspended in the air, hold my weight. I lay there watching the ropes, convinced that at any second I would smash to the hard ground below with a thud. I was lying in a hammock but my heart pounded with catastrophic anxiety.

I knew it was ridiculous, that I needed to get over myself. That I was a very first world problem. Believe me, I beat myself up about that good and proper. But I couldn't. A quote from *Paradise Lost* went round and round in my brain. 'The mind is its own place, and in itself/ Can make a heav'n of hell, a hell of heav'n.' It was apt; I was simultaneously in paradise and the darkest place.

Yet that day would have a significance, a long-term resonance even, that while I was enduring it I could not comprehend. For it was on that unlikely day that I lit a spark, a tiny flame, that would light the way forward, like the white dot of hope in the middle of the black in the Yin-Yang symbol.

I gave up fighting demons in my hammock and swam out into the bay instead – aiming to get right round a lone boat that was moored way out beyond the break. As I struck out around the anchor, a blonde head poked out from under the sail. She looked to be in her mid-fifties. She said her name was Nancy, and then she and the man next to her smiled and invited me aboard. As I dripped onto their deck and we drank beer, she told me, in that frank and open way holiday acquaintants often do, how they'd ended up living on that boat in a remote part of Jamaica's south coast.

Nancy and Billy, her partner, had known each other since they were three years old. When Nancy separated from her husband after twenty years and three children, she and Billy reconnected, pooled all their savings – around $20,000 – and bought the cheapest boat they could find, from a down-at-heel marina in Puerto Rico. Living at sea was not always the easiest; the boat was small, they were at the mercy of the weather and the tides, and sometimes, she admitted, she wanted 'to throw Billy and myself off the bloody thing'. But what chimed with me that day and lit the spark that has stayed with me ever since was Nancy's pure joy in her midlife adventure.

Together they had sailed from Puerto Rico to Antigua, from St Vincent to Grenada. They decided to hunker down for hurricane season in Trinidad, but to get there meant crossing a part of the Caribbean famous for pirates. 'We turned off our lights and radar and sailed blind to Trinidad to avoid the attentions of pirates. When it was land ho and we saw pelicans and dolphins and smelt the earth I was filled with gratitude.'

In the intensity of living at sea and the constant moving on and change, Nancy discovered what she calls 'resonance'. Resonance is a fascinating metric for evaluating your life. 'It's when the outside of your life finally fits with the interior,' she explained. 'By that I mean the outside fits with how you feel on the inside. The two are finally in harmony. When we finally speak our truths, when we admit them to ourselves, then we can design a life for ourselves which mirrors what really turns us on. That is living in true resonance.

'I meet so many women who live in dissonance. They have an internal sense of themselves, where their deepest longings live, their deepest truths – what I call their truthiest truths – that they rarely, if ever, speak out loud. Many women don't express their true desires or show their real nature even to themselves. It gets filed under "impossible" before it is even spoken.'

That felt so immediately right to me. Nancy's experience, her bravery in setting out to create the life that was right for her, that filled her with joy, not only gave me hope in that moment that I could do the same, but provided a kind of road map of what it might look like. It was a window into understanding how so many of us can reach fifty and realise the life that we have worked so hard to craft and create doesn't serve the truthiest truth of who we really are. That if we are truly going to feel fulfilled as we age then some massive aspects of ourselves and our lives are going to have to change.

Some of us have that change thrust upon us; others call it in. But whether we summon it or it happens to us, the truth is that the majority of us experience huge life shifts at this point. But there isn't much out there to guide us through this midlife maelstrom, or much discussion of how this change feels or what it can look like. That was one of the sparks for this book, my Noon community and my journey. To paint that new landscape, to articulate what a midlife transformation might look like.

'This time of life is an invitation,' explained Nancy. 'But that invitation does not always show up benignly. Sometimes we get kicked closer to our goal. That can be painful. For me that kicking was a psychotic breakdown after my divorce. The result of having been adopted at birth, of having never dealt with that initial trauma, that massive rejection. For others in midlife it is redundancy, or cancer, or betrayal, or a death of a person or of what has defined us.

'Tuning in to ourselves is about slowing down, noticing how things feel in our bodies, what hurts – rather than numbing that with food, or busyness or booze or whatever else, we need to really notice how we are feeling. To do the work means noticing the deep longing and acting on it, even if it is difficult. We will be taken to our knees but we will rise up again. There will be an annihilation of what we were which will clear space for what and who we really want to be.'

There was something about Nancy, about her honesty, her adventure, her joy, her lived experience of reinvention after a kicking, which lit that same flame in me. When she asked me about myself, what might make my own life resonant, I articulated for the first time the dream that I had of changing the story that we tell about the later stages of women's lives to something more positive. How I had the germ of an idea to start a community for women in midlife to help bring about for them just the kind of resonant transformation that she had accomplished. To create a new map of what this next stage in a woman's life might look like.

That day, on that boat, was the first time I had spoken out loud about my dream to start a platform, a movement to empower women in midlife. It was the seed of the idea that eventually became Noon – and out of Noon, this book.

Secret: What is your truthiest truth? What would you dare to do if you weren't afraid? I spoke my new purpose on that boat. I didn't know it then, but it was the start of my own new chapter. In the dark of that day ignited the spark of my journey to find a life that reflects the truthiest truth of the real me.

Saying yes to joy

What do you love? What reliably makes you happy? Where do you find joy? For me the answer is water – swimming, preferably. But watching waves crash against rocks, or just sun on water, or a flowing river will also do. I'd rather be in it, though. When I was a kid I was called 'the Fish', and they could never get me out of a swimming pool; I'd glide around for hours, mostly underwater. I never got sick of it. It felt like my own special, weightless world. In water I felt free, graceful, at peace.

So when I suddenly had a lot more time in my life I started to swim every day in a pond near my house. I started in summer and just carried on all through the winter. I found that whatever else was happening, the minutes I spent in the water always had a revivifying effect. They made me feel better.

The path to the pond winds through a grove of horse chestnut trees, their high vivid green canopy is like a natural cathedral. As I walk through, I intentionally look up, I listen to the birdsong, I breathe more deeply. I turn off my phone and am totally there, in the present, in the moment.

I go every day at noon. Sometimes I meet friends, particularly a new friend, Hannah. She calls me her 'Burnout Big Sister': we met shortly after she left the company she founded because she had nothing left to give. Our daily cold swims have been therapy for us both.

The Ladies' Pond is home to a kind of self-appointed sisterhood, a community in the midst of the city. An oasis. For me it has formed

the backdrop to these last three years of change. I know it intimately.
It has taught me to take notice of the changing seasons, the way bare
branches give way to buds, then blossom, green leaves, red leaves and
then brown twigs again. I've also learnt to look out for my friends,
both human and not – Hannah, sure, but also the heron, and the fox
and, on rare days of high good fortune, a pair of kingfishers who zoom
over my swimming head. Their iridescent blue feathers streak above
the undulating green surface of the water; a fleeting spark of joy and
good fortune. An invitation. A promise. Blink and you miss them.

One hot day I was breast-stroking towards the back of the pond,
willow tree swaying overhead, the reeds high to my right – think Millais'
painting of Ophelia – when I saw a snake. I watched it for a beat or two
before realising what it was. It came scooting across the pond, fast –
like the top of a brown stick. At first, I wondered if it was the head of
a cormorant, bird body hidden below the dark water. Or if it was a weird
fish, with a raised head. But then it came closer and I could see its long
serpent body shimmying speedily in S-shapes under the surface. I'd
never seen a snake in the pond, or even heard of the possibility of one
being there. Though, I remembered that a few weeks before, a grass
snake had slithered across my path in an adjacent meadow.

Both times I surprised myself. I've always been scared of snakes;
okay, truth, I'm borderline phobic. I went to a hen do once where
a friend wrapped a white python round her pregnant stomach; I was
so revolted I had to leave the room.

But I seem to have changed. Rather than being scared by the snake in
the pond, I was intrigued. I did get a fear frisson, a shiver of adrenaline,
but it swiftly morphed into a sensation of curiosity at this wondrous,
strange, genuinely new experience (there aren't too many of those at
fifty!). And again, when the snake appeared on the path, I'd initially
jumped, but then had the strangest sense that it was trying to tell me
something.

It would have been anathema to my hard-headed hack former self, but I have come to think that an up-close encounter with a wild creature has meaning. It's as if the universe is trying to tell us something. The great psychologist and thinker Carl Jung referred to such encounters as 'psychopomps'. A psychopomp is a mediator between the conscious and unconscious realms, personified as a wise man or woman or sometimes a helpful or unexpected animal. Digging further, I discovered that the sudden appearance of a snake in your life signifies inner transformation, shifts, the shedding of skins and the divine feminine (Eve anyone?). But coupled with water, the snake's transformational qualities are magnified; a snake in water is emblematic of huge renewal and healing.

The next day I saw Hannah swimming towards me as I launched myself off the jetty – and she was sad. She'd been dumped by a good friend and just couldn't get her head around why, or accept that there really was no way to fix it. The grief that accompanies such a rupture, how our good friends both sustain and define us (and how losing one cuts us to the core), is rarely spoken of. But it is another kind of bereavement. Particularly when the friend is deeply woven into our lives, part of its very warp and weft. Hannah said she was trying to practise 'letting go' of the friend and the grief. I said I thought 'letting go' was a deeply unhelpful phrase. It had come up at one of the Noon Circles I run, where Queenagers share their midlife collisions, and we'd all agreed that it makes shedding a big part of your life sound as easy as letting a satin ribbon slip gently through your fingers. In my experience that kind of 'letting go' is more akin to having a limb chopped off, without anaesthetic! It is more like being pruned; having your now extraneous tendrils, once loved and carefully grown, hacked off with an axe.

Such a pruning is painful, and sad; bits of you are ripped away. It hurts. You want them back. It's brutal. But with time, as all gardeners know, strong green shoots grow back where the old rotten bits were ossifying. The pruning strips us back to our essence, to where the sap is still flowing, to where we can regrow and even thrive. We don't 'get over it', instead the loss becomes part of our warp and weft. We regrow around that scar.

In the Noon Circles we often talk about the battle for acceptance. How hard it is to accept that a beloved spouse is dead and not coming back. Or has left us or that we don't love them anymore. Or that we've been made redundant. That an old friendship is finished. That we will never have children. Or that our children no longer need us; that they have grown and flown. Some acceptances are harder than others.

I've learnt that one way to start seeing the new shape of your life, particularly when it is frighteningly in flux, is to intentionally lean into the sense of overwhelming uncertainty.

What does that mean in practice? For me it meant consciously summoning in and sitting with the unknown and its accompanying anxiety. Really letting it in and looking it straight in the face. Let me explain. When I was at my most panicky about what the future might hold, I could feel the fear about the uncertainty of what was to come pulsating through my body. Literally pulsing, like a fever. This was particularly acute when I had Covid, right at the beginning of the pandemic. I was feeling anxious anyway – but add to that the contagious terror of a disease which at that time was killing people and it was not easy. My body was already throbbing, with a high temperature. At one point it was so bad I begged my husband to turn off the washing machine downstairs, which I assumed was what was vibrating the bed. Turned out it wasn't even running; it was my own fever making me shake. I haven't had to be sponged down to lower my temperature like that since I was a child. I'm sure the fact that I was at a low ebb and felt like the stuffing had been knocked out of me made the Covid symptoms worse. I was flat out in bed for three weeks and weak even after that.

Back then, the TV made my head ache – and the news was full of woe – so I started listening to podcasts and then audiobooks. It was during this freefall time when I was stalked by constant dread and anxiety that I remembered an old colleague – Chris Evans, the British

radio DJ – telling me about the book *The Power of Now* and how helpful
he had found it. I looked it up. It was by a German guy called Eckhart
Tolle. I selected it on my phone and began listening to his soporific
Germanic voice extolling the virtues of being right here, right now.
He explained how most of what we worry about has already happened
(regret) or hasn't happened yet (anxiety about the future). That if we
just concentrate on being where we are, the sun on our face, the leaves
waving outside, the buzz of a fly, even me lying there feeling rough in
my bed – everything is actually fine. And that, being okay here in the
now, in this present moment, is actually all that matters. Ultimately, the
endless stream of 'now' is all that we have, so we might as well learn to
enjoy it rather than constantly worrying about the past or the future.
He explained that meditation was a way to inhabit that 'now' moment.

I had never meditated before in my life. The very idea of me doing
so would make most people who knew me hoot with laughter. I was
someone who never sat still, was rarely quiet and never stopped. I'd
had no time in my hectic schedule for meditation.

But extreme times called for extreme measures, and sitting there
listening to Eckhart I was literally shaking with panic about the past
and the future. I felt like I had nothing to lose – something had to give.
I also thought it might help. So I sat up in bed, closed my eyes and just
started quietly breathing in and out.

Quite quickly, I began to notice colours dancing behind my eyelids.
A deep purple, sometimes green or yellow too. It felt peaceful. I would
summon up the way that the golden sunlight came through the dappled
branches of the trees at the pond. Or a particular memory of the sea
at sunset, the inside of a wave illuminated by rays of light. I created
a simple mantra for myself: 'Golden light. Golden light.' (Since then
I've embraced Vietnamese monk Thich Nhat Hanh's mantra, from his
brilliant book *Breathe, You Are Alive*: 'Breathing in, I know I am alive.
Breathing out, I smile to life.' It is simple yet effective. Indeed, Thich
Nhat teaches how fear keeps us focused on the past or worried about the

future, but that if we can acknowledge our fear, we can realise that right now we are okay, that here today we are still alive and our bodies are working marvellously, which is the ancient Buddhist wisdom Eckhart Tolle drew upon.)

I started doing twenty minutes like this every day in the morning just after I woke up, before I even looked at my phone. I still do. It has become an essential part of my new life.

At the end of my morning meditation session when I was feeling at my calmest, I would intentionally summon in the uncertainty, visualising breathing the unknown into the back of my heart. Welcoming it as it swirled around my body. Looking the fear straight in the eye.

Everything in my life was in flux. Change was happening. The uncertainty was real; I had no idea what was to come, what the future would look like. By summoning the uncertainty in and welcoming it – rather than resisting it or hiding from it – I had a sense of almost floating on the unknown, resting on the change like lying on a lilo along a flowing river. Letting it carry me. When I surrendered to the fact that I couldn't control what was to come, that it was all up in the air and way bigger than me, I began to sense that inside that scary, massive question mark about the future there also lurked a sense of newness, of possibility, of hope. (As well as the terror and panic.)

Essentially, if everything is in flux, there is no point in pretending it isn't. And when you stop and think about it, change is the only thing we can ever be completely certain of. Change is evidence of life unfolding. After all, when we really break it down, we are tiny organic, living specks on a blue planet spinning fast in endless space. Everything is changing all the time; in fact, it is probably a kind of madness to think that anything will ever stay the same, or that we have control over any of it. Realising that, accepting that uncertainty was my new normal, was a huge relief.

But for me, that first shift – learning to allow in the change, to sit with the flux, to surf on the uncertainty, to move towards what felt frightening and unknown rather than blocking it out – became a crucial tool in learning to manage the huge transition in my life.

As the future has felt less scary and some of the things I dreamt of (and summoned in) have begun to manifest – running retreats, writing a Queenager book, building a community of midlife women and a business – I've found myself doing less intentional welcoming of the unknown. I'd kind of got out of the habit. But weirdly, the day before I saw the snake, I had actively done it again as part of a group meditation.

And later that same day I'd had a transformational conversation with Jaqueline Sussman in America, who practises a new kind of therapeutic method with many female leaders in Silicon Valley, called Eidetic Imaging. It is based on the latest neuroscience about how our brains store images, and how the minutiae of the pictures in our minds – for instance the exact pictures we summon if, say, we think of being at home with our parents when we were small – reveal huge amounts about the emotional context, and baggage, that we carry with us.

I asked Sussman to give me an eidetics exercise to do with her over Zoom so I could experience it rather than just being told the theory. She asked me to picture my mother and father in my head. Just the first images that surfaced of them from when I was a kid. I saw a picture in my mind of my father trying to cook a pork chop stew in a terracotta pot. I hadn't thought of that memory forever; it isn't from a photograph. It hails from a time when my parents had just separated and my dad had taken me and my two siblings (I was five, they were three and eighteen months) away for the weekend by himself. He'd never cooked anything before; but he was trying. I remember him calling my grandmother to ask her for advice, looking perplexed at the folds of white pork fat.

Sussman asked me about my mother. She wanted me to switch the images of my two parents over, so a different one was on the left and right. It was hard. My mother didn't want to budge. And then finally she did and suddenly I felt a huge rush of paternal love; like a sluice gate opening, or a river bursting its banks. In the aftermath of my parents' divorce I had very much been in my mother's camp. The eidetics technique of shifting around these images in my mind had unleashed a tsunami of love from my father which I had never been able to feel before, I just hadn't been able to access it. And suddenly, while I was on this Zoom call with a woman I had never met, this wave of love sloshed in, accompanied by a host of new loving memories of my father which until that moment I had lost or blanked out. It was very emotional but also felt profoundly right. As though I finally had access to a whole heap of emotional ballast that had always been missing. I realised that not being able to access my father's love before had caused me to be permanently out of balance. Wobbly.

I wept then and for several hours that afternoon, not out of sadness but out of a deep gratitude for all that had always been there but which until that moment I could not feel. That love from my dad made me feel so different, like my internal compass had shifted to where it was supposed to be. It made me feel solid in a way I never had before. Whole. It felt like a significant step on this long journey, this reckoning with everything that I am at this point in my life.

And then the next morning I saw the snake swimming in the pond. With all its connotations of transformation, inner healing, the shedding of past personas, of the skins that no longer serve us. It was like the universe saying: 'Look! See! Believe! Change is possible.'

And then there was Hannah, still sad about her friend. Stuck on it, ruminating; the way we get when something that has anchored us, defined us, goes and the rupture leaves us reeling. She couldn't understand why she wasn't able to just move on, let it go …

We talked about the snake, and acceptance and change and about control. Hannah is a powerful woman, a woman who founded a movement, who knows she has agency in the world. But the truth is that when it comes to others, we have no control. We have to relinquish rowing the boat and let ourselves float on the great river of chance and uncertainty; truly surrender to the unknown.

We got out of the pond and shared a tearful, soggy hug on the jetty.

What I have learnt is that for each of us, the stepping stones – the way across the river of uncertainty to what is to come next in our lives – are found in accepting and welcoming in the unknown and then in finding our joy. Seeking out what makes us feel most alive, most in flow, most ourselves, and doing more of that. If we start there, with what makes us feel good, we have a good chance of success.

For me, I followed the joy that I found in water and swimming and it has led me to so much renewal, friendship and revelation. That simple decision to go to the pond every day has allowed me to feel part of something larger than myself and to let that work its magic.

Secret: Say yes to joy in your life – follow its stepping stones and it will take you to a better version of yourself.

Forged in fire

It was a glorious, sunny summer evening as we headed down a secret path below Clifton Suspension Bridge. The city of Bristol was spread out behind us in all its pastel-coloured glory. The tidal waters lapped at the side of a pontoon surrounded by houseboats. As I teetered carefully down the jetty in my high heels and best frock, a family of ducks quacked past.

The stage was set for a riverside Queenager wedding; my mate Sophie, sixty-two, was tying the knot for the third time to her new love, Ben, sixty-five. Of course such nuptials are rather more complicated than when the protagonists are in their twenties; inevitably, after so much life, we all come with baggage. And it would be fair to say that this pair came with more than most! My friend has a son from her first marriage and a daughter, who had a baby of her own when she was only eighteen. The groom also had several offspring but on this glorious evening it was a picture of a happy blended family – and the happy couple wore the biggest grins of all.

Sophie more than anyone I've ever met exemplifies the findings of the Noon research around Queenagers being forged in fire. Essentially, the survey – the largest study of its kind ever undertaken in the UK – found that by the time we hit fifty, over half of women (aged 45–60) had been through at least five massive life events. These included divorce, bereavement, redundancy, bankruptcy, health issues, mental health troubles, domestic abuse, elderly parents needing support, a teenage child with an illness or other complications. Whenever I reel off that list when I am doing public speaking I see heads nodding in silent ticks – yes, yes, yes – like a kind of Queenager bingo!

But it's not all gloom and doom. By far the most surprising – and uplifting – part of the research was that those who had been through the most, were now the happiest. Why? Because having been through the midlife maelstrom they'd now got their lives set up just the way they wanted. One woman talked about being 'delightedly divorced'. Another, a celebrant in the Midlands, said that despite losing her job and having bowel cancer she'd 'found in the aftermath a new happiness, I love my work, I feel lucky to be alive – every day is like a gift'. One of the women spoke about 'the wisdom in the room – it comes from experience of having been through it all, and survived'. Another said: 'I keep saying to myself – don't do something stupid like walk out in front of a bus. I've just got this life business sussed! I'm just getting going.'

Sophie put it to me in a different way: 'I only know a couple of people who have had no major traumas and I feel a bit like they are living life in two dimensions, or only in black and white. Everything I have been through makes all the good things that much better, even the small ones. Every Tuesday Ben and I change the sheets and we get into crisp, fresh-smelling linen together and that makes me so happy. Or a good cup of tea….' She trails off, smiling.

If anyone deserves a happy new chapter it is Sophie. Talk about troubles coming not in singles but battalions. She has had, as she puts it, 'the full-on midlife clusterfuck!' That is why it was so joyous for those of us who love her to see her beaming in her beautiful wedding dress, a beacon of happiness and Queenager possibility. She is living proof that there really is much more to come, inspiration for when we are at our lowest ebb. It certainly felt like that to me, that day, when I was deep in my own funk.

Sophie was married young and she and her husband drifted apart – amicably – towards the end of her twenties. Her second marriage began in a whirlwind of romance. Her husband was swish and rich; her life seemed a whirlwind of sophisticated weekends in Paris and being whisked off to swanky hotels around the globe. She already had a son, and was delighted when she got pregnant again and gave birth to a daughter, Alex. But her rather self-centred husband didn't take that well to family life and before Alex was in her teens he'd run off with a much younger woman. I remember having lunch with Sophie during that time and barely recognising the woman I thought I knew, her face distorted with grief, baggy with tears and betrayal. It got worse. Alex began to bunk off school. Soon Sophie got her first call from the police: 'We've got your daughter here at the station, she's been smoking weed and hanging out with people she shouldn't. Please come and get her.' That was the start of a long, scary road.

Alex had problems with her mental health – she was referred for treatment but it didn't seem to help. She began to self-harm. She'd disappear from home, and Sophie would have no idea where she was. And then Alex got a boyfriend; he was bad news. Sophie had a stark choice: to ban her daughter's boyfriend from the house or not see her daughter. 'Everyone thought I was mad. There was total craziness going on, but I knew it was the only way I could keep any kind of stability or oversight of my daughter.'

All this time Alex was out of control, despite Sophie's best efforts. At one point Sophie didn't see her for months. 'She was a child who thought she knew everything.' And then, just when Sophie thought it couldn't get any worse, Alex got pregnant. She was still a teenager. 'Suddenly there was an army of social workers involved. I thought a termination would be best for everyone but I also knew it wasn't my place to advise her. It was her choice.'

Alex decided to keep the baby. 'It was a high-risk strategy, the most high-risk strategy of all. She was a child herself and now she was becoming a mother. My house was like the set of *Only Fools and Horses*, a cast of all sorts of pretty insalubrious characters. I couldn't bring any of my friends back to my house – I was ashamed of what my home life had become – but I also couldn't defenestrate my daughter.'

There were dark times. 'I came back home once to discover Alex had thrown all of my clothes out of the window into the front garden because I'd refused to give her any money because she hadn't done the washing-up. I had to operate some serious tough love. It was so hard.

'I was in my late fifties, all my friends were beginning to be free, beginning to be Queenagers, and I was faced with either having to adopt my own grandchild or see her taken into care if Alex didn't sort herself out.'

Miraculously, Alex dug deep and did just that. 'She was a spectacularly good mum; as a little girl she'd loved puppies and kittens, she was always super-caring. That just came back to the fore. She loved her daughter and realised she was going to lose her if she didn't change, so she did. Having the child was the making of her. The reset her life and brain needed. It was high stakes but it worked.'

Sophie's face is glowing with pride as she tells me how Alex did an access course and got her education back on track, eventually getting into university and gaining a degree in law so she could help the kinds of lost boys she had got to know in her teens. And just as Alex began to get her life back together, Sophie met Ben. 'We knew each other as acquaintances. There was a party I went to every summer where he would always be. Even though everyone was quite tipsy, it's weird I remember every one of our conversations and so does he.'

Ben had been through his own bad divorce and also had a child with mental health issues. 'He was one of the only people I'd met who understood a bit what I had been through with Alex. It was a very slow, old-fashioned courtship. We were both so wary.'

Ben's post-divorce project was fitting out a knackered old Mustang in his garage. Sophie's house was not far away. 'I started popping down to chat to him while he was working. Or he'd come and see me for a drink at the end of the day. I was so lonely and mistrustful after what had happened with my former husband. Both of us were so terrified of jumping into anything. When I was younger I'd always leapt first and worried later when it came to relationships. This was the opposite. We circled around each other until we were totally sure. It's funny, we've talked about it and we don't know if we'd have been together if we'd met earlier in our lives. We've had to grow into the people we've become.'

Eventually they got together. Alex and the baby lived with them for a while. 'It was the most beautiful thing, the two of them. At first Alex was like a feral cat but Ben just hung in there. He took us all on: me, Alex, my granddaughter, warts and all. He has been like the father she never had.

'Now it just feels like bliss, the greatest happiness of my life. And you know what I think the best moment was, when I finally felt it would all be okay? It was the first time Ben came to stay at my house on a Saturday night and we spent the whole of Sunday just lying in bed drinking coffee and reading the papers. I realised that what I had most missed was not having someone to do something with, but someone to do *nothing* with. That intimate witness who cares what you had for lunch.'

I truly believe that Sophie and Ben's wedding was one of the happiest I have ever seen. Alex and her gorgeous daughter smiled and hung out with Ben's kids. In the midst of Sophie's troubles, it seemed impossible that Alex could turn it around, or that Sophie could mend her heart, broken by betrayal, and find a new man. But with time and love and patience her life turned around. Sophie's story for me beautifully encompasses that rarely discussed trajectory of hitting the rocks in midlife but coming through healed, stronger, happier. We saw it in our research – that midlife is not a crisis, as the cliché goes, but a chrysalis. That the more women go through the more likely they are to have shed the things that no longer serve them and to have their lives set up exactly as they want them. Being forged in fire helps them become the women they always wanted to be. Sophie told me her story because she wants every Queenager having a midlife clusterfuck to know that it can get better. That there is always the possibility of a happy ending!

I understand that urge. She is right that in our lowest times we can lose that hope, lose the capacity to believe in ourselves and our resurrection. I know I did. But Sophie's story shows that if we keep believing, keep going, believe that the sun will shine again, then we can come through and be happy once more. She is the proof. And you can be too!

Secret: Queenagers are forged in fire – that's what creates their strength and wisdom and is the basis of great future happiness. All the suffering only makes the good things when they return all the sweeter.

Shapeshifting

I truly feel that now, at fifty-two, I am – for the first time in my life – slowly becoming more and more myself. That feels like a nuts sentence to write after five full decades on this earth. Who else have I been if not me for all that time? Have I not inhabited my own body, made my own decisions? The answer is yes ... But! In our Noon research half the women agreed with the statement that fifty 'is when it is finally all about me, when I return to my own dreams, my own ambitions after years of putting everyone else first'.

But why does it take so long for us to become our true selves, the women we always wanted to be? Well, as women particularly, we are moulded by the prevailing culture to put other people's needs higher than our own. Just think of the women around you: we look after our kids, our partners, our employees, our pets. Too often we come bottom of our own to-do lists. I was so busy just getting through my rammed days, coping with the demands of the job and my family, that it was only when I got booted out that I even paused to ask myself *why* I was doing it, *who* it was serving.

At the paper where I worked I'd always felt like a square peg in a round hole, a leftie on a right-wing title, a woman in a sea of macho men. But I'd grown up in a family where achievement was everything, where you only existed if you could point to a power title or a big accomplishment (it's not by accident that four of my mum's five children went to Oxford University; it was drummed into us to achieve). In fact, when I got made redundant and I called my mother to tell her what had happened, the first thing she said to me was, 'You will miss the power and the prestige.' Not, 'You poor darling, everything will be all right.' But, 'You'll miss the power and the prestige …'

Ouch!

In some ways the brutality and directness of that comment were helpful. It stung like hell, but it gave me clarity. It helped me see some of the pressures that had kept me going in such a high-profile role for so long. My own insecurities about whether I was good enough, plus the family spur to keep achieving, very publicly, was strong. Yet when, after being whacked, I put that gold-embossed cloak which signified external power and status down, I felt loss, sure, but also, after the initial sadness and shock, an unexpected sense of freedom. Once I had taken it off, I realised that the cloak was heavy, bulky, cumbersome. That it had forced me to act for decades in ways that weren't truly me.

Often in my old life, if I am honest, I would consult my own inner compass and realise that the job required me to do or say the exact opposite of my own instincts. It was exhausting always having to second-guess myself, to fit my decisions and opinions to someone else's view of what was right. Especially as usually that someone was an older, more powerful man. I spent two decades serving the needs of my bosses and the newspaper, driven by an urge to succeed, to achieve, as I had been trained to do by both my upbringing and education.

It was an exciting, fast-paced but brutal world; I'd grown extra armour – literally – to protect me. After I left the paper, I lost several stone. Not intentionally, I wasn't dieting, the weight just fell off me like I didn't need that extra buffer, that armouring layer, to protect the inner me anymore. The real me, which was softer, and vulnerable – nothing like the one I was expected to project. Newspapers are all about being first to the scoop, hitting the deadline, competition. The pressure was always on to do better. It was a swashbuckling place, where you showed weakness at your peril. Going in to see some of the bosses was like being in a cage with a tiger; I never let my guard down. Inevitably, with the benefit of hindsight, I regret some of the things I did; the role and that world required a toughness that was not always kind. I am sorry for the hurt I caused to those around me. As I have worked through my own numbness since – with many different activities, some of which I document in this book – I realised I'd caused colleagues pain, that the cloak I wore cast a shadow. It has been a bitter pill to see and understand that retrospectively. I am sorrier than I can say. I hope I am now a gentler, kinder version of my former self. I certainly try to be.

Losing that cloak hurt. But I can see now that the shedding of that identity was both painful and necessary. To begin with I had a sense of being an outcast. I had recurring dreams of trying to enter my old office and being turned away by security, or of going down the familiar corridor only for it to lead me into a maze of blockades and tunnels where I got lost. But as the shock receded and the weeks passed, I began to realise there were definite upsides to my new life. That without that heavy black *Game of Thrones*-style power cloak, accessorised with its weighty gold and fur, I was lighter and more nimble; liberated in fact. That without it, I could write my own rules, paddle my own canoe – that, at fifty, for the first time in my life, I could be my own person and express *my* truth. That I was finally free to please myself – not my family, or my boss, or anyone else. It was like I'd spent a lifetime ticking other people's boxes, living out ideas of success I had had thrust upon me. I realised that now I was free to follow my own instincts and define success for myself.

The shift out of that mindset wasn't easy. Releasing my own true voice from its inner cage was terrifying. The editor lurking in the back of my brain kept screaming that it wasn't safe to break all the codes I'd lived by for so long, to expose my true self and opinions.

Every time I wrote something that my old self wouldn't have been allowed to express, it felt terrifying to put it live. I literally shook with fear.

Many people have said to me that they envy the ease with which I put my voice out into the world, that they find doing the same incredibly hard. Well, the truth is, it *is* hard. Hard for me, hard for all women; our freedom of expression comes with danger and pain. I felt it as a physical constriction in my throat. That isn't stupid. It is only a few centuries since women in the UK and Europe were burnt at the stake as witches for speaking out, for speaking truth, for living in a way that challenged social mores. Deep inside us the cultural conditioning screams 'Danger!' when we start to say things that challenge the status quo. I'll come back to the effect of that programming on us all later in the book.

But finally allowing myself to follow my instincts has reaped huge rewards. During the last three years I have found that the more I have leant into expressing my true views even when they have made me vulnerable – or maybe particularly when they have made me vulnerable – the more connection I have made with my community and with women on the same path. 'I don't know how you do it but every week you just seem to say what I've been thinking,' said one of my Queenagers at one of our get-togethers. Those kinds of comments make it all worthwhile.

I haven't been able to do this on my own. I have done it with the support of some great Queenagers – many on the Noon Advisory Board and many who have been through a similar midlife resurrection. One of the people who have given me huge insight and strength on this mission is Kati Taunt, a trauma therapist and friend. She and I have spent many hours, often under canvas, or walking through woods or on the Ridgeway or other ancient British paths, sharing and bouncing around our concerns and observations; she from the perspective of her therapeutic practice, where she comes alongside to support many

Queenagers. Me from this journey – and both of us from treading our own paths through huge midlife transition. Mine initially professional but which turned into a major life re-evaluation; and hers more personal – a divorce, an ill older child – which have also forced big life changes.

So here is Kati's therapeutic theory and story of this shapeshifting we do in midlife: why it takes us so long to get here – and why it does not come without pain and pushback.

'Queenagers are emerging from years of intense career-shaping, home-building, in many cases parenting too, and they all harbour a similar underlying discombobulation of restlessness coupled with uncertainty about the shape of their future,' Kati explains. 'Often they present with depression or anxiety, challenges around marriage breakdown, or bereavement, redundancy or empty nests, but there is also something deeper going on. The women have an intuitive sense that the shape they have been holding for so many years no longer fits. It feels itchy or baggy – dragging or constricting. Or just not a shape which is really true to them anymore.'

Kati explains that we force ourselves into the shapes that our parents want us to be; that as children and beyond we often contort ourselves so that our carers respond favourably to us, so that they keep us safe. That is of course entirely sensible in evolutionary terms, particularly when we are small and vulnerable.

'We take the shape that gets rewarded with love, affection and care. The shape that means we are not hurt, or put in danger, or rejected.' Of course, all of us are 'socialised' as children. 'That means things as basic as manners, being taught as a child to share or say please, to be socially acceptable so that we are liked by others and learn to succeed at life. These are necessary, of course, but we also need to take notice of what we had done to us, how we were forced to take the shapes we have, and what we are passing on to our children.'

One of her clients, she says, is a midlife woman who learnt to suppress her own contagious enthusiasm for life so as not to over-whelm her depressive husband and to keep their family unit intact for the children. Another creates a false self when her mother comes to visit. She not only bakes a cake and makes everyone sit down for tea (something that never happens otherwise) but insists that her teenagers take off their goth make-up and black clothes and dress in a way their granny approves of. 'In this way this woman is shifting her shape in front of her mother to avoid the familiar disapproval, attack and shaming, even though she is fifty!' For Queenagers the judgements of our mothers – raised in a time when women had fewer choices, when attracting and keeping a man was paramount – can be particularly harsh. In one Noon Circle a woman spoke about how, when she told her mother she was pregnant, she'd responded: 'Don't expect me to look after the little bastard.' Another said that when she called her mother to say that her husband had left, leaving her with two tiny children, her mother replied: 'What did you do?' The need to screen ourselves from such criticisms is all too evident.

And it is not just our mothers. Kati also points to a female CEO who engages in high-energy blokeish banter with her male colleagues even though she is naturally quiet, so that 'she is seen as an equal, part of the chaps' club'. Our generation of women has been socialised into being people pleasers, often putting everyone else's needs above our own.

Kati insists that we shouldn't blame ourselves for this shapeshifting. 'Throughout our lives, when we are faced with the choice between *authenticity* (doing what our impulse drives us to be, i.e. being the shape where our energy most naturally takes us) or *attachment* (being kept safe and getting our needs met, not rocking the boat), we tend to choose attachment. We opt to hold the shape that others want us to be in, because by doing so we get relationships, careers, families, friendships and safety. We are programmed like this to do society's bidding.'

In some ways, Kati says, we are all being a bit like Barbapapa and

Barbamama in the 1970s cartoon series – those bright-coloured blobs that morphed into useful shapes to fit in difficult spots.

'So with Queenagers I now frame my thinking in terms of the shift that would help them find a new, more authentic, shape. The one they would flow into if they were encouraged to be truly themselves and could slough off all that conditioning.'

This insight from Kati so resonates with me, both in terms of my own shapeshifting and what I see when I sit in the Noon Circle. So many women admit they have spent so long contorting themselves into what they think the world/their boss/their partner wants them to be, or what they have been taught to want to be by the media, or what their parents wanted them to be, that they have forgotten, or buried, who they truly are or what they might authentically become. One woman said to me: 'I don't understand how I got here. I look at my life and I feel like I didn't choose any of it. I don't want any of it. That I've forgotten who I really am and don't know how I got here.' Often, when the women realise this about themselves they weep. Often, they don't even know how to start refinding themselves, let alone have any idea what their final true shape might be.

So what helps?

I reckon the first step to finding your true shape is to remember what you like, to reconnect with what brings you joy – and to build some of it into your life. Think about the things that bring you joy as being like stepping stones to your true authentic self. Remembering one thing you love, or used to love, or want to do, or wanted to do, often reminds you of another – just giving yourself some time and space to tune in to your own desires rather than other people's is a good place to start. It could be listening to music *you* choose no matter what anyone around you thinks of it. I realised I spent my entire time listening to songs chosen by my husband or daughters. It felt both awakening and empowering to get my own speaker and create my own soundtrack to my life again. Others get back in touch with themselves by taking up a hobby they've always fancied, or picking up an instrument they haven't played for years, or going on a trip somewhere meaningful to them.

Kati says that within the therapeutic process she 'asks the women to gently look at all the times they compromised their authenticity and shaped their life-force energy into roles and shapes for others and for their own survival'.

Kati says it is like standing 'together in front of a magnificent dressing-up box of the costumes which fitted former shapes or roles. Together we take them out and talk about them: some costumes we say goodbye to fondly, others, which have been constricting, or painful, or bad, we consign to the bin. Then I ask what costume or shape they would choose for themselves.'

It is not a sudden process. It takes time to become our new selves. 'I suggest they take their new shape on a spin out into the world, listening to their impulses, noticing when they take a shape particularly because it allows them to fit in, especially with parents or family. Those old patterns are hard to shift until we become conscious of what we are doing, and then we can stop.'

Of course, the world won't always like our new shape. Kati warns her Queenagers that there are reasons why we contorted ourselves, so when we stop doing it, the people around us often try to force us back into the jigsaw piece, or shape, we've rejected. That is entirely normal. 'If the shape you were in was functional to the system it evolved in, expect others to try to push you back into it. Just notice that. Good luck!'

She is right – both about the need to shapeshift in midlife and how those around us often don't want us to change. Just take my mother. As Kati said when I first told her what my mum had said when I was whacked: 'Projection.' It was my mother who was going to miss the power and the prestige. It was contorting myself into the shape which suited her that had kept me in that heavy power cloak for so long. Sorry, Mum. But I'm fifty and it's my life. And you know what? I am so much happier, kinder and freer without it!

Secret: What could your new shape look like? Who or what in your life is forcing you to take a shape which isn't the one you would authentically choose? Is it time to shapeshift anyway? Why not give it a try.

Finding a new tribe

It's a rainy May bank holiday Monday. The lushness of the green of the unfurling leaves and the blue froth of bluebells sing against the lowering grey sky as I walk to the pond for my daily swim. It's been quite the week for contrasts. I've just returned from leading our first ever Noon Tour; me and twelve Queenagers, accompanied by two female guides, trekked 75 kilometres in four days, through ravines and over mountains, by gushing rivers full of snowmelt and poppy-filled fields of wheat. We were in the High Atlas mountains in Morocco, seven hours from Marrakesh in the Valley of the Roses, which were being fragrantly harvested by hand all around us.

The giddying chasm between normal London life – filled with stuff, technology, excess – compared to the stripped-back life we led on the trek has made me ponder. For eight days we lived like the locals of the Atlas. Rooms had no furniture, so we sat on mats on the floor, close together, passing plates and glasses down the line, sharing simple platters of vegetables and couscous – the small rooms, or courtyards, alive with laughter. We sang and danced with drums and claps – uproariously. Often there was one loo, one shower between all fifteen of us. No one complained. We shared, and accommodated each other. We slept under the stars. I didn't hear a single cross word. In that simplicity we gained such richness.

And the laughter; we giggled and cackled, guffawed and belly-laughed. It was a core workout to make a Pilates teacher proud. I laughed so much my stomach hurt. The kind of uncontrollable, heaving mirth that takes only a fleeting catch of another's eye to start you off again, wheezing with shared hilarity. The best of times.

They say laughter is the best medicine – I would agree. Particularly when coupled with biblical scenery – red rocks reminiscent of Utah, Uluru or the Grand Canyon. The immensity of the mountains, the glare of the sun, the tweeting of birds, the soft steps of fifteen women walking as one up hill and down dale.

We began as strangers, really. Seven days later we were all firm friends.

I write and talk often about the benefits of finding a new crew in midlife – how being with a group who don't know you as a colleague, or a wife, or mother, or friend, who have no preconceptions about what or who you are, what you like, what you can do, is immensely liberating. Indeed, I would even say that that kind of blank canvas, or new community, is a necessary crutch for starting a new chapter; for trying out what you might or could become.

Well, this trip provided the perfect blank canvas. We arrived tired and jaded. Strangers. Many of the women were wan with care; bearing the burdens of bereavement, or caring for partners or children in trouble, weighed down by many demands – single motherhood, big jobs, that sense that Covid has shrunk our worlds, loss of confidence, previous ill health … the full Queenager gamut.

But as we walked and bonded all that receded: 'The wonderful thing about this trip is that no one has wanted anything from me,' said one woman. 'I have felt totally free, to be me, to let it all go, to talk about myself, to go deep, to explore and dream – and to laugh, of course.'

As the days passed by and the kilometres clocked up, we all began to shed the loads we'd been carrying. Complexions brightened, years fell off, as the emotional baggage was shed, big decisions made. (One woman decided to close her business, another to marry her partner, another to leave her relationship.) New ways forward became clear where once they had felt impossible. Some were habitual trekkers; some had never been on an off-grid journey like this before. 'I haven't climbed a mountain for twenty years,' said one Queenager. 'I'd forgotten the exhilaration of looking down on creation.' It was heady to be beyond roads. Out of phone range. Living in these mountains, walking the goatherds' paths with our nomad guides, Mama Bia and Sara, as people have done here for centuries.

When one of us faltered – and, oh yes, there were tears – the group rallied round to support; maybe with an energy-boosting sweet, a Compeed plaster, a bear hug, an understanding squeeze of the arm or an empathetic look. The group switched around, we all walked with everyone; sharing our deepest secrets, our hopes, our fears. There was often a cry of: 'There are people who have known me for thirty years who don't know any of this stuff.'

We were all processing, talking it out. In that endless, biblical landscape everything seemed clearer. Water brings green and life – terraced fields by the snowmelt rivers throbbed with poppies and wheat, roses and fecundity, families working together ploughing with mules, or weeding. In families who all live in one room, conjugal relations occur when wives bring lunch to their husbands in the field. Those fields were fertile in all senses!

But beyond the reach of the water there was just sand and rock. Timeless, vast, scoured by wind. In that wildness we felt small. There was space for everything, time to talk and reflect. And most importantly, perhaps, to unburden, to just let it all float away on the wind or the river. And throughout, the thud of boots on rocks, the murmur of confidences exchanged, the cackles of exuberant laughter and joie de vivre.

It wasn't luxurious. We lived like Berber nomads. Some nights we slept six to a room – dormitory style, joshing each other about snoring and mess. (I win the prize there; I was put in the corner where my exploding rucksack could be contained.)

We were led by Mama Bia, sixty-one – a true Queenager who became one of Morocco's first female mountain guides at fifty-five; talk about finding your vocation in midlife. She struck a slow but deceptively relentless pace, never faltering as she climbed mountains without breaking sweat in top-to-toe crimson velvet, with thick leggings underneath and woolly socks. Real nomads wear velour – who knew? Just looking at her made me feel hot.

Mama Bia's is a story of hope, of change. Proof that coming into your prime in midlife, being a Queenager, is not just a white Western phenomenon. At fourteen, she was married off to a nomad and had her first child as she walked a 900-kilometre annual circuit from the Sahara to the High Atlas, herding cattle to fresh pastures. Every day her job was to scout for and carry back water to the camp, while her husband and his tribe (in accordance with Berber tradition, she'd had to leave her own family behind not knowing if she would ever see them again) tended to some 5,000 goats.

It was an unhappy time. When I asked her how far she had walked in those years, she shook her head. 'Too far!' she said simply but poignantly. She told us she'd given birth in the wilderness with only her mother-in-law (!) to help – another Berber tradition.

After three years of suffering and loneliness, she returned to her birth family; disgraced, divorced, an outcast. For the next thirty years she eschewed other husbands – 'too much trouble', she told me wryly. (She nodded with approval when she heard that half of our group were divorced … she looked around at them, one by one, smiling at each broadly in shared kinship.)

Once back home, she made a life in her family village, which clings to the rocky terracotta-red walls of the Valley of the Roses gorge. The road only arrived here in 2016, and Mama Bia's village is the end of the line. Her house is made of mud and straw bricks. In her small courtyard she keeps baby goats and lambs, below are her fields where, with water from the river, she grows wheat for couscous and a few staple vegetables. These days she also lives with her two granddaughters, eight and six. Her only son married but the relationship broke down and his wife left; so she is the girls' main carer. When she goes off on treks, the girls stay with Mama Bia's brother, who runs a guesthouse nearby. He describes her as 'crazy' but is proud of her new incarnation as a mountain guide. This came about because Zina Bencheikh, the Moroccan boss of Intrepid Travel, introduced women-only tours and started hiring female guides in 2017. At fifty-five, Mama Bia became one of the first female mountain guides in the country and is now a local celebrity. 'Guiding women's groups has brought me freedom and happiness,' Mama Bia told me, beaming. I smiled back at her. Walking with her, I explained, had brought my Queenagers freedom and happiness, too. We hugged in mutual appreciation. When we got to the top of a steep mountain and she pointed to me and said, 'Eleanor – nomad!' it was one of the best compliments I have ever had.

One morning, schlepping up an 1,800-metre pass surrounded by rocks, cliffs and thyme, we bumped into one of Mama Bia's nomad relatives. The woman with her goats and seven children was temporarily residing (as nomads do and Mama Bia did when she was one of them) in an encampment around a stone hut/barn just off the track we were following. I peered into her tent – a plastic sheet weighed down with rocks, the bed a simple cotton lungi laid over the stony ground. My own thin sleeping mat from the night before suddenly seemed like the bed of kings. We thought Mama Bia might settle down to chat with this long-lost kinswoman – but with the most cursory of nods and a pat on the back, she moved on. A Berber version of 'Later!'

Mama Bia's knowledge infused our trip. As we toiled up the mountains, she would leap about gathering fragrant herbs – rue, thyme, spearmint – and crush them under our noses for energy. At lunch she made us bread, nomad style. Burying the dough in the earth and covering it with hot coals, she stoked it with a blazing juniper bush. For shelter from the sun, she guided us into an ancient nomad cave, like something out of Jean M. Auel's *The Mammoth Hunters*. 'Here,' she said, 'there is always wind.' She was right. The noon sun was baking, but outside the cave a breeze blew off the mountain, cooling the hot flanks of the mules who rested in the patchy shade of a gnarled juniper bush. Mama Bia's people have been living here like this for millennia.

It was humbling to get her perspective. In one village she pointed out the adult graveyard; about forty rocks which marked the burial mounds. A few steps further on there was another: this one littered with ten times as many rock headstones. It was the children's graveyard. 'Berber women are strong; they are not supposed to cry when their babies die. They move near the fire, where if their eyes water they can blame it on the smoke,' she said. Looking at all that loss in the parched ground, I cried.

Mama Bia pushed us. Sitting with her at the top of the highest pass, the folds of the mountains rippling below us on and on, the Sahara beyond, she gave me a rare hug. I felt exultant, full of Queenager energy.

Half an hour later, 21 kilometres in, feet aching, on a scree-covered path littered with large rocks from recent storms, I crashed. 'How much further?' I asked. 'Two and a half hours – maybe more,' said Mama Bia. I pushed back. Her timeline was not acceptable. 'I thought we were nearly there?' I whined. She shook her head. I realised that trying to push back on the timeline was ludicrous. This wasn't a negotiation. It was a path. A mountain. It would take as long as it took, no matter how tired I was or how much I wanted it to be shorter. Mama Bia's eyes twinkled at me. She told us to keep our eyes on the ground and watch our feet. 'No selfies!'

We made it down. Eventually!

After 23 kilometres we reached our spartan guesthouse and collapsed gratefully on its terrace, legs throbbing, triumphant at having endured. We drank mint tea and lolled on mats looking over the verdant river valley, chatting while Mama Bia, Sara and our hostesses for the night decorated our hands and feet lovingly with henna (it is not just for beauty, it has antiseptic properties and protects the hands when working in the fields).

In the morning my right foot was so sore I could only stand on tiptoe. Mama Bia grabbed it: for five agonising minutes she grinded and brutally massaged my Achilles tendon, while I screamed in pain. Miraculously, when I stood up afterwards, I could walk ... Nomad magic.

That day we had to ford and re-ford a river. The current was strong. Alone we could have been whisked away. Together we were indomitable. Under Mama Bia's gaze we formed a Queenager wall, holding onto each other's arms in an interlinked chain of bodies facing the river; stronger together, strong enough to cross safely with Mama Bia showing the way. It was a good metaphor for the trip. When one faltered, the others had her back. We formed a loving unit – a truly safe space.

Back in Marrakesh we went to the hammam. Moroccan women go once a week; a rare place they meet to chat outside the home. What is said in the hammam, stays in the hammam. It is run by a phalanx of strong women, who lay you on a mat and scrub you all (and I mean *all*) over. I haven't been washed like that by another woman since I was a child. It was curiously moving; sensual yet functional – not sexual. The breasts of the 'queen of the hammam' dropped down to her knees, she rinsed all of our crevices, saw all of our secrets – even lifting the flap of my stomach so she could wash underneath it. We laughed so hard we thought we might get evicted. It was a fitting way to end the trip. Clean, scrubbed – they kept pointing to the 'spaghetti' of dirt they'd scoured out of our skin – reborn.

I can't remember the last time I laughed so much, shared so much, witnessed so much beauty or so much change. I truly believe that when women support women, we can do anything, be anything, help each other into an amazing next chapter. This week in Morocco I saw that in action. It was beautiful, moving, special. Proof that we are not done – that, as Mama Bia shows, there is as the Noon motto goes: So Much More to Come.

Secret: Stripping back our lives to the basics, living simply, engaging with others, remembering what we love are the stepping stones that lead us out of the darkness into the light. Those small spots of joy are the light to a happier way of being in the world. When we follow them – they show us the way.

PART TWO

LOVE AND RELATIONSHIPS

What do I know about love? For me, love is rocklike – modest, enduring, steadfast. It is like a promontory sticking out into the sea, penetrated by ripples of water, heated by sun, lashed by wind, buffeted by storms. But if we keep the faith, if we hang in there, we'll be blessed with glorious sunsets and bright new dawns, feel the ecstatic touch of frothing foam as it penetrates the whole of us. We'll know that new things are growing within and without us.

I have found that love comes to us in strange forms – it won't necessarily be what or where we expect. But when it comes, like the sun, it illuminates everything, inside and out, and makes our lives whole. To love also means to be there for those we care about, offering our love and support just because we feel it. Because we want to. Offering our love as the best and purest part of ourselves, seeking no reward.

This section is all about love and the relationships which sustain us. Around 40 per cent of Queenagers at this point in their lives are on their own. Indeed, so many couples split up in their fifties and sixties that they even have their own moniker: silver splitters. We'll be delving into the dos and don'ts of divorce, how to renegotiate a long-term relationship to avoid that outcome (if at all possible), alongside how to date again in midlife.

For some of us, midlife is the point at which we embrace a new partner, possibly even of a new sex. And some of us choose to leave our partners – which comes with its own brand of heartache. Of course negotiating relationships, particularly new ones, comes with a side-order of the gendered ageism and various other forms of prejudice in our society. What is it like to be a Sikh divorcee? Why might a Muslim woman consider becoming someone's second wife? Love at this stage comes in many forms, and for many of us the love of old and new friends can be the most enduring love of all.

But I want to begin this section by exploring the truth about long-term relationships. They often get a bad rap when it comes to romance – Ester Perel talks about 'mating in captivity', the challenge of keeping lust alive in the marital bed. We've all heard the jokes about the husband who says he only gets sex once a year and, when asked why he looks so happy, grins and says: 'Tonight's the night!' But it's not all gloom and doom. Given this is a book about midlife and the majority of us are married or cohabiting (sixty per cent according to our Noon research), I thought I'd kick off with a rare upbeat account of a relationship of nearly three decades' standing: my own.

It was my twentieth wedding anniversary and I was supposed to be off having a lovely time at the Manoir aux Quat'Saisons, the hotel where we spent the night before our wedding. But instead I am at home; my husband got Covid and is confined to quarters. So I am being nurse instead. It's made me realise how much he does: the fridge is bare, the washing is piling up. I had to go and get my eldest daughter back from uni and managed to smash her cafetière and knock her appallingly packed stuff off the trolley onto the quad. She kept saying, 'We need Dad.' She was right.

I never thought I would get married – it didn't rank highly for me as an institution, perhaps because I had attended both my parents' second weddings before I was ten. I wore white carnations in my hair and a turquoise green frock when Mum married my stepfather Peter.

He was a rock; when I woke up in the night it was he who interpreted my dreams (he was a psychoanalyst). When I went to teenage parties he'd pick me up; grumpy, sat in a grey Saab Turbo listening to Radio 4. But always reliably there. However late it was.

I didn't have much luck with boyfriends till I met my husband. I picked wrong 'uns – didn't really understand what good looked like until I went to India to visit an old uni pal, who introduced me to Derek. I spend a lot of time talking to Queenagers who want to meet someone. Well, sometimes that person just walks into our lives. When I met Derek, I was lying reading a book on the roof of the Shanti Guest House in Hampi, Karnataka – an ancient city, full of deserted temples – in a landscape that looks like gods have been throwing boulders around for larks. 'Meet Derek,' said my travel buddy. I looked up and there he was. He had long hair, a noble Velasquez-style face, and was wearing a yellow T-shirt (which is weird, he never wears yellow). He'd just been walking the Annapurna circuit in Nepal. He'd also studied English Literature at uni, like me. We had a chat. He came down to my room for some shade and a smoke. We kept on chatting … and I suppose we've never stopped.

The mates I was travelling with wanted to chat up girls and drink fizzy beer – it was a dry city; all booze came in on a motorbike over bumpy roads – they weren't interested in exploring the temples with me. Derek was. We bought oranges and cheese, tomatoes and bread, and went on endless picnics and forays round the old ruins. I remember reaching out to take a bag of oranges from his hand one morning and he flinched when I touched him. I knew in that second there was a spark between us, that he felt it too: electric. Those days were golden. We wandered through temples with marble pillars that played tunes, saw snakes under rocks, hung out in the Mango Tree Restaurant on a bend in the river where food ordered at 11am would arrive at 4pm (they had to go and shop for it and make it in a leisurely manner – kofta takes time). We'd lounge in hammocks, talking nonsense. One night Derek purloined some fire clubs and juggled flames for me. I was in.

After three weeks I returned to London. I was twenty-six and features editor on the *Telegraph*. Derek was heading to Bodh Gaya to do a retreat where Buddha found enlightenment, and setting off again into the Himalayas to walk some more. We wrote to each other, my letters sent poste restante to random post offices in the mountains – Paharganj, Naggar, Rishikesh. I didn't know if he'd received them or not. But I got his. I still have them – packed carefully in a special box with my children's baby teeth. Treasures. Pearls beyond price.

Right from the start, Derek made me feel different – a nicer, calmer version of myself. He was a moral compass. He also had my back. Always. Years later, I remember going to an antenatal yoga class where we had to fall back into the arms of our partner. I have never been a sylph – and I was enormously pregnant – but I knew he had me, that he would catch me no matter what.

Those of us who grow up being the responsible ones, the grown-ups, even when we were actually the children, crave that certainty, that security, the knowledge that someone else is looking out for you. That it's not, always, all down to you. That someone else can share the load. He was the first person who made me feel like that: safe. Looked after. I just knew this relationship was different. My friends were suspicious – 'A juggler? You met in India? Really? Are you sure?' But I *knew* he was the right one for me.

I've given that advice to so many people over the years – don't choose your partner for your friends, or your family; choose the person who is right for you. The one who sets you on fire, who makes you feel safe and is your best friend. It doesn't matter what anyone else thinks; *you* know. Be brave. I've made some bad decisions in my life, but choosing and being chosen by Derek was the best one I ever made. Unlikely on paper, but right.

We got married in Oxford Register Office with only two guests, our two witnesses – my brother Max (the son of my stepfather, the other rock in my life; I wanted his name on my marriage certificate) and Liz, Derek's best friend. I suppose it was fitting that my daughter was also at the wedding, albeit in my stomach. I cried all the way through the ceremony. I blamed my bump for my tears. Said being pregnant had made me uncontrollably emotional. But that wasn't the real reason. I cried because I felt so moved and happy and relieved – like I'd finally come home. Marrying Derek is the best thing I ever did. This summer I found myself wearing the dress I got married in (it is light green, Ghost, satin) – it is as if time has come full circle. All those elements that were there twenty years ago – the friends, the daughter, the dress, the husband – are still very present in my life, two decades on (albeit older and wrinklier).

So I suppose this story is about circularity, but also about certainty. Those rare certainties we have in life when big love creeps in and makes your soul its home. Writing this it occurs to me that perhaps it is fitting that I have spent the week of our anniversary looking after Derek as he has spent so much of our life together looking after me. Maybe me running up- and downstairs with meals and paracetamol, mopping his brow, is a more appropriate way to celebrate all our years together than a fancy night at a posh hotel. It has certainly been a lesson in appreciation. And it's made me realise that I can go and do lovely things with friends and my gorgeous daughters – but it's not the same without him. That with no Derek there is a big piece missing.

I got Covid twice, so did the girls, but Derek never caught it, even though he nursed me – and them – through two bouts. How strange that he should end up sick now.

What are those wedding vows? 'For better, for worse, for richer, for poorer, in sickness and in health.' In marriage you take the rough with the smooth. And sometimes in the rough you find the smooth; it is in the cherishing of each other that you find the gold.

Renegotiating our relationships

'Love is not love which alters when it alteration finds,' wrote Shakespeare. I'd beg to differ. Even the best, most loving partnerships require a bit of renegotiation from time to time. A wise therapist told me that all of her patients in midlife, if they are to stay together and avoid becoming part of the silver-splitter statistics (couples over fifty these days are the most likely to get divorced), come to a new reckoning about how things might work if they are to continue on together.

The relationship therapist said that every marriage, or long-term partnership, needs renegotiating at least once a year. And if you've been together a long time then a big reckoning, where you talk honestly about what is and isn't working and what you really need, is a must. He said that so many of his patients arrived with the same complaint: their partners seemed to expend mega effort on their careers, their friends, their bosses, their colleagues, their hobbies, their elderly parents, even their children and pets, but the person who most often came bottom of their list, or certainly felt that they did, was their supposed beloved.

'How is it,' the therapist asked, 'that we kick off in our relationships with that jittery feeling of love and rainbows, our significant other rocks our world, we'll do anything for them ... and then we get married to them, or move in together, and a decade or so later they are the person to whom we make the least effort? They are the one who gets the knackered, grumpy, in-your-tracksuit-and-passing-out version of you ... never the shiny, excited one.'

I thought about my own marriage – twenty-seven years together, over two decades since we tied the knot. And myself, how often do I put my husband at the top of my endless to-do list? The answer is from now on I am going to make sure he is there more.

These days there seems to be divorce all around me – friends parting ways, hooking up with new people. Some looking cheerful, others devastated. Children in the mix. I know what that's like – my parents split up when I was five. I remember Tom Jones being asked how his marriage had survived four decades of showbiz: 'Just don't get divorced!' he'd quipped. There's something in that. But we also know that midlife is the peak time for divorce. Often the kids leave home and two strangers look at each other across the breakfast table and think, Hmmm, is this it? If I've got twenty or thirty more years – do I want to spend it with you?

This is where that renegotiation malarkey comes in. My stepfather Peter Hildebrand wrote a book called *Beyond Midlife Crisis* – it was all about the huge psychological development that people are capable of in later life. How we think we are formed, have become who we are after fifty years on the planet, but that the truth is we can always learn, and change – and the reality in his clinical practice (he was a psychoanalyst and the head of the Adult Department at the Tavistock Clinic, so he'd seen a few patients!) was that people made massive shifts and often became far happier as they aged. This has been proved: the economist David Blanchflower has demonstrated there is a U-curve of happiness, peaking in our younger lives, declining to the age of forty-seven – and then coming right back up again as we get older.

But back to that therapist. He was talking about the importance of valuing your partner (which sounds obvious but is hard in practice) and renegotiating our roles. I see it all around me: one woman I know said to her husband that they could stay together but she wanted to spend three months of every year painting in Spain. Another's husband said he was devoted to cycling (a true Mamil, or middle-aged man in

Lycra) and wanted to go off on frequent cycling tours – and the woman responded by saying great, she wanted to retrain as a teacher. They are both happy and have new creative outlets.

At one of our Noon Circles a Queenager was telling me how her husband, having worked in an office all his life, has taken early retirement and is for the first time ever doing the family shop, taking the cat to the vet and ferrying their son to cricket matches – he wants constantly to tell her all about it in minute detail when she is trying to work and look after her ageing mother. 'It drives me nuts,' she says. 'I've been working and doing all of that domestic stuff for years and he was never interested, but now he is doing it I am supposed to keep up a constant litany of how marvellous he is for doing it. I'm grateful, but FFS!'

It is often the small things in relationships that are the dealbreakers. Does your partner think of you when they go shopping, buy the things you like? When you are stressed, can they make you smile? I was super-stressed out about a speech the other day so my husband dressed up in my new trouser suit with a frizzy blonde wig and got one of my daughters to photograph him in it. He sent the message just before he knew I was going on stage: I laughed so much I forgot to be nervous.

Maybe we should remind ourselves that there are many kinds of love; do you know about *agape*, the Greek word for a love that is not erotic and romantic but kind, nurturing and cherishing? The kindness of picking up your partner's socks, or cooking their favourite meal. Love comes in many forms but at the root of all of them is consideration – sometimes putting someone else's needs or feelings above our own.

But by the time they hit fifty many women have had their fill of that; it came out clearly in our research that Queenagers see these years as *their* time, to revisit their own dreams, have time for themselves. Indeed, our Noon research found that time for themselves was more important than partner, the job they love, friends or an active sex life.

But sometimes there is a less radical solution to finding that freedom. Maybe rather than splitting with our partners, we can renegotiate?

Of course, there are some relationships which cannot be saved. Divorce is increasingly common for those of us in midlife, so who better to advise us than Sandra Davis of Mishcon de Reya, one of the world's top divorce lawyers, and the woman Diana, Princess of Wales turned to when she separated from Prince Charles and who advised Jerry Hall when she separated from Mick Jagger. I went to meet Sandra in her sleek offices in central London, where she told me that more women than men initiate divorce proceedings, but that they are 'not usually the motivators for the split. They come to see me because their husband has had an affair, or is exhibiting controlling behaviour or psychological abuse. It's rarely physical abuse. For the most part women are far more tolerant of abusive behaviour than you might expect.'

Sandra deals primarily with high net worth and ultra-high net worth separations, where the rules can be a bit different – but her thirty years of negotiating the messy fallout of marriages has given her insights that are valuable for the rest of us too. Her prime piece of advice is to avoid getting divorced if at all possible.

'A divorce upends all relationships, not just the one with the spouse,' she warns. 'It affects family, friends, colleagues; it will alter forever your relationship with your children's grandparents.' So often, she says, women are so angry that they 'don't think through the social and psychological consequences of a split with enough care. Dissolving a marriage, particularly a long-term one, is a painful process, don't underestimate what it will involve. Divorce is like a train crash. *Smash.* Never do it lightly.'

She says that the first thing she encourages a prospective client to do is always to try to resolve any issues. 'It's generally a lot easier to manage problems in a marriage or around a separation in a practical, consensual way. If you're entirely selfish about it, if you operate on the one-life theory – you know, "I'm not happy … I'll just throw away this tissue, chuck it out and have another one" – you are in for a shock. Divorce doesn't work like that. Occasionally it works like that for men, but it isn't like that for women. Particularly for Queenagers.'

The chilling reality, she explains, is that the majority of her midlife women who are divorcing end up on their own with their support network of female friends. We met because she was interested in the community I was building as she knew how crucial it could be for her clients and others in the same situation. In her experience it can prove harder for Queenagers to find another mate. I am frequently struck by the often-indecent haste with which male divorcees or widowers find someone else to take their ex-spouse's place – is that because women are choosier, I wonder, while men just want someone to fill that role?

Sandra's take is that the kind of men she is dealing with 'can often choose to be with a woman half his age, start again, have more kids and never be judged for it. It's the age-old trade-off – money, status, power and a younger female. It's getting slightly easier for women to be with younger men but it's still not as common.'

Could that be because the kind of women who are coming to her are the ones who have got into relationships in the first place because of that kind of dynamic? That they were always trophy wives and so get traded in for a younger model?

Sandra shakes her head. 'I don't think so,' she says and there is a pause. I get a hint of the kind of steel that has made her such a fearsome advocate for her clients. 'Often the women who I see have been in the marriage a long time. They've started out in a relatively equal deal and money has been made during their partnership. With the Queenagers, I find that often the wife has not worked, even if she had a successful career beforehand; she's looked after the family, so she's become de-skilled in the workplace, and therefore lost confidence and become more dependent. And so it's much harder for her to re-establish herself as a middle-aged woman going back into the workplace after, say, a twenty-five-year break.'

We discussed this imbalance of power at an event we did together. I talked about the number of my female contemporaries – bright Oxbridge women – who married their university peers and then found their own career ambitions trumped by a super-successful husband whose extreme job required her to pick up the domestic slack. Sandra's key piece of advice was for women to keep up their own income stream and independence, and a separate bank account. The stories of women bamboozled over money by their husbands hiding assets and lying to the court were heartbreaking. Some of the women were genuinely terrified by what their husbands might do when they sought a divorce; manifestly, the most dangerous time for a woman leaving an abusive relationship is when she says she is going.

Given Sandra's long – grisly – experience of humanity during divorce, her tips for what to do if this is something you are considering are valuable:

'Get your house in order. Understand your finances, work out what you spend, what you need, how much things cost; ask yourself what the future will look like if your husband's not there, you lose everything that goes with being a couple. What will you do? Don't be naive about what it will mean to be "free" – remember, divorce is a bit like indigestion, you don't get rid of your spouse, they keep revisiting you like acid reflux.'

This is particularly true if there are children involved. As a child of divorce myself I second Sandra's advice to keep things as amicable as possible from the beginning, to always behave with dignity and try, as much as humanly possible, to embody Michelle Obama's maxim, first uttered during her speech at the Democratic National Convention in 2016: 'When they go low, we go high.' It is agonisingly difficult, of course, but it is important to play the long game, even if a former spouse is bad-mouthing you. 'You are going to have to go on co-parenting, so the less bitterness there is the better. Be kind. When you are tempted to go nuclear, or be unreasonable, look long and hard at a picture of your children. Ask yourself: what will happen to the kids, where will they live, who will have custody, how will it work for them? Your ex will be there at every parents' evening, or wedding … forever.'

It sounds chastening but Sandra counsels that it may well *not* be better on the other side. That new love who seems so perfect? Hmmm, the divorce rate for second marriages is even higher than for first because of the added burden of blended families. And as Sandra says, 'You take yourself and all your baggage into the next marriage too.'

It is telling that a woman who has been so intimately involved in divorce is so keen to advise against it. 'Why are you contemplating divorce?' she asks. 'Have you tried counselling, couples therapy, solution-focused mediation which might enable you to think about this in a different way. Could you renegotiate your relationship in a way that might work for you? Are you putting too much weight on this relationship, have you tried other ways to make yourself happier, such as a new interest or career? Could you find a new tribe of people to hang out with, or something else to do that would make you happier inside the marriage?'

Sandra insists: 'The grass isn't greener; one in four people who separate wish they had never divorced and over half regret it.'

I say that a Queenager friend of mine had described her own divorce as 'like a depth charge – it just goes on blowing things up, down and down, triggering every sadness and every insecurity, blowing up every part of your life'. Sandra agrees.

'Many of the women I see say their friends expect them just to get over it and move on, negating the wound they have from the breakdown of what has been decades of their life. They expect the wound to close over, for it to get better, but I see that they can get re-triggered at any point.' She sighs. I know what she means. There are some huge challenges we go through in midlife that are too big for our friends; where we need to pull in more specialist help: a divorce coach, a therapist, group sessions like those we run at Noon for women divorcing where they can get support from those who have been through it. Sometimes, however much we love our friends and however supportive they are, our midlife clusterfuck needs more help to be thrown at it to get us through. There is no shame in that.

'I think what's really absent for this set of divorcees is connectivity, meeting other women like them who are in the same boat. The most important thing is being with other women who understand, who can shed some light, share some knowledge.'

Secret: Divorce only as a last resort, when there really is no help of salvation – and build yourself a supportive cocoon of experts and those who have been through it to support you. However lovely your friends are, some life crises are too much for them to bear. It is hard to ask for help, but being vulnerable enough to ask and then to accept the support offered is the way we get through hard times.

When things don't go right, go left

The nuggets of wisdom we need to get us out of a bad place and into something better are often found – in my experience – in the granularity of the details of other people's stories of change. When I left my big job and found myself in the wilderness of wondering what would come next, I discovered that being with others who had either sought change, or also experienced it happening to them, was a great balm. It was a ski instructor who had left a career in the City after a breakdown and burnout who told me: 'When things aren't going right, it is time to turn left.' It's a bit management speak but there is concentrated wisdom in that. He is right – the definition of madness is to go on doing the same thing and expect a different outcome. The bravery is in admitting we have got to the end of the line – and knowing it is time to take a new direction, a new path.

Taking time out of normal life to go on a retreat, to be somewhere new, with a new crew, to try out a new version of myself was massively important for me in being able to think about my life and future differently. Those few days out of life allow us a safe zone in which to shapeshift; to road test a new way of being in the world. Change is difficult, for sure. What I sought were tales of the granularity of how change happens. I got so tired of superficial stories along the lines of: one day I was working in a bank, now look at me, I'm a crofter in Scotland. I craved the details of the shift. What exactly living in a new way, going left when it wasn't going right, starting a totally new kind of life, felt and looked like.

After I left the paper, a friend of a friend mentioned a retreat she'd been on at a fabulous house in Yorkshire, surrounded by dales and woods and beauty. I was looking for my own version of that 'left' turn, so I went.

I remember driving up to that imposing house in the dark, alone, full of doubt and sadness, wondering why on earth I had gone, what I was doing there. I was used to being plunged into strange situations; it is what you do as a journalist. And yet this time I wasn't there to observe, but to take part. My panic only intensified the next morning when we were marched up a hill, through a wood, to a large stone arch.

'As you walk through it,' the retreat leader said, 'shout out what you want to leave behind and what you want to bring into your life.'

What did I want? The question alone was a facer. If I was honest, in essence I wanted not to feel miserable and rejected; to have a purpose again. The others began to take their turns, stepping through the arch into their new lives, as instructed, calling out what they wanted them to be. I felt a shiver of cringe. Could I do this? It not only felt stupid but exposing. I had a word with myself: change happens when you do something different, try something new. None of these people knew anything about me; I wasn't going to be popping up in *Private Eye* anymore. There was a huge freedom in the anonymity of this new tribe, an unfamiliar freedom from expectation or judgement.

I took a deep breath and walked through the arch. 'I embrace the unknown, a new chapter, a new me. I accept that the past is the past and there is no way back!' I shouted.

It felt good to say it out loud. Next, I took off my shoes and walked on the wet grass, following a spiral of stones into and then out of the centre. The earth felt squishy and moist but not unpleasant under my bare feet. In front of me a woman trod the same path, others were already returning and as we passed each other we smiled. Each of us on our own journey, winding into the middle of the labyrinth, then out again … alone, but together, with companions. The metaphor of walking one's own path, but not alone, was made manifest. It was so simple but it felt reassuring, even profound.

As I walked, quietly, in my mind I began to leaf back through the last few years – in the rare moments when I'd had time to stop to think, I knew I was stale. Each week felt like a Groundhog Day treadmill. The same calendar of meetings on the same days at the same times. My life had become rigid, predictable. The same people, many of whom I had worked with for fifteen or twenty years. It was as hard as ever to get great stories, big interviews, but the impact of anything we printed was far less than it had been in the heyday of newspapers. Our influence was massively waning, and it no longer felt like the industry I'd joined. I'd known on some level that I needed a change. Friends had been saying to me for a while that I should move on. But I didn't have the courage to jump out of my big power job myself. Now the universe had certainly sent change to me!

I looked around me and found to my surprise that I felt pleased to be right here, right now. I sensed for the first time, deep and small, the very first feelings of relief, of escape. That just maybe, beyond the very real feelings of rejection, humiliation and being cast out from my tribe and the life I had known, there could be an upside. That maybe, just like that labyrinth that wound in and out, I would find a new path. A new direction, left, not right. That it was time. That it could even be good!

Later that day I sat in a circle and listened to the others as they explained what had brought them here too. One story in particular resonated with me and the sense I had of being forced to take a new direction. Jennifer was already further down the path.

She explained that she had separated from her husband and was now on her own with her teenage daughter at fifty-two. The revelation which changed her life had come during a drink on one of those glorious English summer evenings. 'The sun was slanting through my pint glass, illuminating the honeysuckle in the garden. I felt expansive and happy. Ha!

'My now-ex looked at me sadly. So sadly that I shivered. I downed my pint and said, "Okay, give it to me straight." I thought he was going to say he'd had an affair. I wish that was all it had been ...'

She looked so sad as she said this that I felt a quiver of emotion going through me too.

'He told me he'd been gambling. I knew he liked a bet – on the horses, the footie. His mates all did it. I tried to laugh it off. He took my arm ... Turned out it was way worse. Not a joke. I started asking him how much: 10k? 20k, 30k, 50k? He kept just shaking his head, burying his face in his hands. I remember my heart starting to race, thinking about our mortgage, our house, our daughter, our *life*. The life I'd worked so hard for.'

She stopped.

'He'd lost over £100k – way more than I earned in a year. Enough that we were going to have to sell our house and even then we'd be in debt that there would be no way out of.'

Jennifer had had to re-evaluate everything: ditch the gym, cancel the Netflix, forget the expensive wine. 'I realised I'd got a bit spoilt, used to nice holidays and meals out. Those days were done. After growing up frugally, I'd thought we were sorted. My husband and I both had professional jobs, we had two kids in private school, a mortgage. I thought my financial fate was sealed; that each year would bring more savings, swelling pensions and eventually a comfortable retirement, rocking chairs optional.' The bitterness in her tone took me back.

For months she'd tried to hold the marriage together, with counselling, support from both families, personal loans. But more financial and mental strain followed. 'As the pressure piled on, I became angrier and more short-tempered. Discussions about the future ended with us standing in the kitchen screaming at one another.'

Throughout he kept promising he'd quit gambling. 'At some point, I stopped believing him. I was suffocating. I felt that if I wanted a future for myself and my child, I had to get out. He was beyond our help ...

Money stuff is weird,' she said. 'More shameful than just being cheated on. I felt stupid. Like a mug, like I should have known. I mourned my smart haircuts and all the other trappings, but most of all I missed the life I'd had: a husband I trusted and relied on, a family, days when money wasn't a constant fear and I didn't wake up wondering, "What will become of us?"'

It's all too common for women to find themselves in this situation after a divorce. A man's income can increase by up to 25 per cent after separation, while women are often plunged into penury. Jennifer described how it had all come to a head one night. 'I was driving and someone pulled out suddenly into the lane in front of me. I yelled a string of obscene words, surprising myself, and then screamed – a long shrill noise that bounced off the windscreen. When it stopped, I screamed again. I felt nothing. I wondered if I was cracking up. That night I cried and cried until eventually I just said: I give up.'

She gave a hollow laugh.

'I wasn't giving up on life. But I realised in that moment that I had to give up my old way of thinking. Everything had changed, forever. There was no way back to my old life, or my old life plan. I realised the only way forward was for me to change too. In a movie this would be when the music would swell as I realised that the true wealth I have is my love for my daughter. But it wasn't that simple. I found that having my world implode was enlightening, for sure, but not in the way movies tell you. There's nothing noble about undergoing a crisis that has you wondering how to afford groceries or a place for your family to live.

'I realised that if I want a new kind of financial situation I'll have to fight for it. I have totally stopped splashing cash on little things we "deserved" like takeaways. Now I only spend money on things which are important in the long term, like my daughter, or a pension.'

Her voice took on a new seriousness. 'And yet, there is something hopeful about this new mindset. It's made me realise that I can completely reimagine my life. If everything *has* to change, then things really *can* change. I've realised I could move to the beach and spend my weekends surfing, or live cheaply and just focus on writing, or start a third-act career which generates loads of cash. Maybe I'll do all of these, or maybe something I have not yet imagined. But this massive shake-up has made me realise that I really can do anything…'

I was blown away by Jennifer's hard-won hope – her realisation that in the death of something old, in the space which that leaves, something new and different and possibly wonderful and completely other than what she had once expected could grow, or be manifested. It was a timely lesson for me in the possibility of reinvention. That out of the ruins of our expectations, a new kind of future might be possible.

I had felt so hurt and rejected but that week helped me to see that, actually, maybe turning left was okay. That that new direction could even mean that I was moving into a better phase. Jennifer's courage and her message that the collapse of everything familiar was actually an opportunity, not just a disaster, made me realise that sometimes something massive has to happen, something has to break, or we have to make the break ourselves, if we are going to shift and change into something better.

Secret: In love and relationships – just as in every other area of our lives – every massive disaster or change carries the seeds of something new. In the space that loss brings, something wonderful can grow if you let it. The transition will be messy, raw and painful but that doesn't mean that there aren't good times ahead. In our Noon research we discovered that the women who had been through the most ended up the happiest. In the clearing that a big loss creates, is space for something new to grow.

Coming out – and finding new love

Right at the very end of my old life, pre-pandemic and before I was removed from my big job, I went to a reception at 10 Downing Street. I've been through that famous black door a few times; to interview British prime ministers David Cameron and Theresa May – but also to parties. However many times you go there, there is always a frisson about entering the nexus of power. That morning Boris Johnson was – ironic, I know – throwing a bash for female journalists. There was a clutch of women's magazine editors (all as glossy as you'd expect), some newspaper hacks like me (scruffier), and Boris's new female ministers looking all keen and corporate in block-colour suits and dresses. The interior of Number 10 is a weird mix of stately-home grand and NHS waiting area; incredible art and portraits of PMs past, but municipal loos with lino floors – everything a bit tatty round the edges.

I spotted my school-gate mate Rose across the room. She and I are veterans of many political party conferences. Interminable weeks where you drink warm white wine in windowless rooms and do speed-dating with politicians and lobbyists (so they can explain policy positions, hoping for favourable coverage, and hacks can get stories). Rose and I always bonded over being what felt like the only non-believers at the Conservative Party Conference. That morning, even from across the room, I could see she looked like the cat who got the cream: radiant. I went over, gave her a hug and said she looked glowing. She pulled me behind a pillar: 'I'm in *love!*' she whispered. I guessed from her giddiness she probably wasn't talking about her husband of several decades. 'Oh my God, Eleanor,' she said. 'I feel reborn, I've never felt like this before. It's, she's … a woman.'

Silver splitters are a global phenomenon. Often when the kids leave home their parents look at each other and go: 'Is this it? Is it you for the rest of my life, and then I die?' – and ring the divorce lawyer. I was desperate to ask Rose for all the details, but it was neither the time nor the place. (Years later she is still blissfully happy, I'm glad to tell you.)

She was by no means the only Queenager to leave her husband for a woman; it is quite the trend! Soon afterwards I met Jo, who told me all about how she'd also left her own marriage for Sarah, whom she'd met on a Woman's March (where else?).

Jo never thought she was the kind of person who would turn out to be gay. She grew up in Yorkshire in a cosy Church of England family, the grumpy, clever one – 'adults called me precocious'. She told me that she had always had a sense of having to rein herself in, a common theme among women with outgoing, exuberant personalities. 'I had a few relationships with men, some nice, a few awful. I enjoyed the flirting but never the sex. I drank heavily all the time. Then friends started getting married and, although every wedding felt not like a beginning, but an ending, I eventually tied the knot too.'

First she was swallowed by the chasm of early years' parenting and then felt herself dissolving into the 'toxic sludge of boredom and resentment'. She ended up with a stay-at-home husband, two children, a four-hour daily commute, persistent headaches and anxiety. 'I could not hide from my own body,' she says.

The day she met Sarah she had arrived early for the Women's March, having negotiated some time away from home to go with a few work friends. 'It was already buzzing, thousands of women smiling in the chilly air. I noticed myself feeling happy. I saw her face through the crowd – grey bob, red lipstick, navy blue anorak. She was part of our group. We carried a home-made sign saying "Feminist as Fuck" and sang "Freedom". She became my best work friend; we'd meet for café lunches, I gave her clothes that didn't fit me anymore. She texted me all the time.'

Then one Sunday evening Sarah rang Jo at home – she usually didn't as she respected the unspoken wall between Jo's family life and her 'Sarah life'. 'Sarah told me she'd got drunk and slept with a woman for the first time. I was both devastated and delighted.'

Jo fought her feelings for Sarah for two years. She even left her job to put some distance between them. It didn't work. 'Being at home was like being underwater, I could hear a new life calling me. Gradually I realised I was going to leave. I didn't know when or if Sarah would be with me when I did. I still hadn't told her, or anyone, how I felt.'

They went out for dinner. Jo got very drunk. She found herself blurting out, 'Everything would have been fine if I hadn't accidentally fallen in love with you.' And that was that. There was no going back.

That was when the real horror started for Jo. 'The telling of the kids, the moving out, the sadmin; marriage is a fucker to undo. But the actual coming out was a total anticlimax. Nobody cares; no one gave two hoots about the gayness. My brother teases me, sure.'

I wanted to know if at some level she had always known that she was attracted to women not men. Jo said she didn't really know, it was hard to say, but admitted that she had always 'fancied Justine Frischmann at school not Damon Albarn. But I married a man. Am I gay now? Yes. Was I always? Probably. Why didn't I see it earlier? Shrugs.'

She still feels guilt about leaving, but 'I don't feel I have to rein myself in anymore. For that I am so grateful.'

I love Jo's story – it is so heartfelt and nuanced, so real. Her joy at finally living the life that is right for her, that feels resonant with who she really is in the core of herself, is so important for all of us to hear. Sure, we're not all going to discover that we were sleeping with the wrong gender all along, but a surprising number of women are finding that their sexuality is more fluid than they thought. That now we are lucky enough to live in a world which is more relaxed about same-sex relationships, we can follow the example of our Gen Z children and broaden our horizons. So – coming out in midlife. It's a thing. If it's your thing – go for it! After all, we only live once … don't waste your precious time here as a sentient being pretending to be something that you are not. Follow your heart!

Secret: The heart wants what the heart wants, and it might surprise you to find it isn't necessarily what it used to be. That's okay. If you want to be happy, don't fight it.

Dating – the dos and don'ts

It was just after 7am when a series of WhatsApps pinged on my phone. 'Please help – I'm being completely ripped off!' It was a Queenager with a high-powered job; she always says she became the managing director her father wanted her to marry – who'd found herself alone at fifty. She didn't mind being single, was sanguine about it. But during the pandemic her only sibling had died suddenly of Covid and her beloved dad had also passed away. 'It was quite a facer to lose half my family in less than a year,' she explained. Whereas before she'd been relaxed about being single because she knew she always had her sister – 'we were a team, I thought we'd grow old together' – she now decided to join one of those super-expensive dating sites which promise the man of your dreams. I'm sorry to say that he had not materialised. This woman is not stupid (far from it) but the site had promised her eight eligible dates over the year and had charged her nearly twenty grand. Now I know that is a fortune, but, as I said, she is a successful lady and, in her own words, 'was just fed up with dating frogs who don't turn into princes, getting buggered about when I am super-busy – and on top of that being sent dick pics'.

Another reason she chose the high-end dating agency was that she was sick of having to downplay her professional success so as not to frighten men off. I can hear you scoffing, really, in 2024? I'm afraid the answer is 'yes'. I've lost count of the number of successful women who lie about how successful/rich/good they are at their jobs until later on in the relationship. I know, depressing. Sigh. (And it is not the only story. At Noon we find that half of women over fifty are the main breadwinner in their family. I personally have always been! But some men haven't yet got the memo…) So yes, she'd spent more than the average wage to join a dating site … and it was a disaster. 'The first date was old enough to be my dad, the second revealed over dinner that he hadn't paid to be on the dating site books at all, which didn't strike me as at all fair', the third 'sounded good on paper but was never in the country'. After that lot, she e-mailed the site asking for her money back – and they refused. Which was why she had contacted me, asking if I would write about it in an attempt to raise the alarm about how rubbish it was.

This is of course quite an extreme example, but the trials and tribulations of Queenager dating are legion. I hear about it a lot from my single friends. The most common scenario is that they start dating someone who says he is extricating himself from his marriage … but several months later it becomes clear that he's not. He's just playing the field, or is only at the beginning of a separation process. Many Queenagers say that the pickings are slim. One told me how she had bumped into an old friend who was the same age as her, and he told her he was on all the dating sites. She said she was surprised, as she hadn't seen him there. Turns out his age parameters were 25–40! He is fifty-five …

But all is not lost. With a doctorate in evolutionary biology, Dr Mairi Macleod is a later-life dating expert with some surprising, science-based, solutions. When I first talked to her, she explained to me that women are hard-wired by our early human ancestry to pick a particular kind of man.

'In our twenties there was such a choice of men. If you fell out of one relationship, you could just fall right into another. Back then the world was our oyster, as I am sure it was yours, too. I was a biologist travelling to remote parts of the planet to study wild monkeys – particularly their sex lives. And also, I have to say, having plenty of sex of my own. What I learnt in my research was that a monkey girl has a lot of the same issues to deal with as we women – picking a good strong father for her babies to help protect them, avoiding or appeasing the males that would try to be controlling and potentially violent, and the odd foray into the forest to seek out new "genetic input" … But one thing female monkeys don't tend to have to endure is ending up on their own in midlife. That's what happened to me.'

When Mairi met her first husband in the late 1990s it was a whirl-wind. 'We stayed at the Ritz, went skiing in Canada, ate at posh res-taurants – he said he wanted everything I did, so when he produced a ring, I said yes. But I'd chosen with my gut instinct rather than my brain, the marriage went tits up very quickly and I had to run for it – although not before I'd managed to have two pregnancies and three babies. When you're on your own with three kids, trogging around the jungle after monkeys is impossible so I took up freelance science journalism. I started writing about human behaviour, particularly sex, attraction and relationships.'

However, once her kids had grown up a bit, she found she was lonely. 'I signed up for some dating sites to find a new man, but it didn't go to plan. I met men and had the odd relationship, but I was making the mistake of following those gut instincts again and getting together with guys who provided the "spark", the "chemistry", but who were no good for the kind of committed, lasting relationship I was looking for as a mum in her late forties. I realised I was done with players, however sexy. I had to evolve the way I was looking for men.'

Mairi realised that evolutionary biology provided the solutions to why we behave, feel, desire and love the way we do.

'I realised that simply following my gut instincts was a road to oblivion – those instincts evolved back in the Stone Age when couplings would have been relatively short term, and brawn and status were all. Nowadays we'd do well to consciously override our evolved instincts and figure out ways to make better relationship decisions that suit us for this stage of life (and the modern world).'

Mairi asked herself what she needed for a happy relationship rather than what she wanted. 'When I met Rob at a singles event, there weren't a million explosions but I liked him.' They got to know each other gradually over a few weeks and he invited her to a ukulele session where he was playing.

'That night I saw a completely different side of Rob, he totally owned the room, he was brilliant, and I really fancied him. I saw him at his best, I found his confidence sweet-spot, and because the desire had grown gradually and we were already compatible and liked each other it became something much more powerful. He's become the real love of my life. But if I'd been following my old ways of looking for men I wouldn't have noticed him.'

Following her own experience, Mairi now runs a business called datingevolved.com to help other Queenagers find their own happy (and we've run seminars with her on Noon). Here are her five tips to help you on your way.

1. Understand the type of man you need

You might want a gorgeous boyfriend, who's six-foot-four with a full head of hair and a salary well into six figures. You might want this kind of man, but so does every other woman – so if you get one of these types, how secure are you going to feel? And chances are he won't have what it takes to make you happy.

I'm not suggesting you 'settle' but I am suggesting you re-prioritise the qualities you're looking for to make sure they're what you need for a happy relationship. I reckon that's a guy who's considerate, trustworthy, and one who'll warm up your side of the bed before you get in.

2. Try a bit of patience

So, you need to suss out what a guy is actually like. Rather than jumping into the sack right away in a firework display, take it slow. If we do get intimate with someone early on, this gets our neurotransmitters going bananas, which then gets us smitten with this guy, even if he turns out not to be a suitable candidate for long-term happiness. Then we spend the next few weeks, or months, or years, trying to get this guy to have the relationship with us that we want, but it's never going to work because he's just not that guy.

Better, then, to approach relationships first as friendships. Identify someone who seems interesting, nice, that you're curious about and would like to get to know better. Who shares your interests, say, in hill walking, or opera, or whatever floats your boat. The science shows that when we get to know someone and we like them, we like their personality, their humour, we then start to find them physically more attractive and we begin to desire them.

So it might not be as exciting as the fireworks guy, but you won't be using up all your emotional energy on someone who's never going to be good for a relationship, and you stand to find a far better bet in the long term.

3. Bite the bullet with online dating

Yes, I know, online dating is no panacea, but it can work and we all know someone who's found love this way. This is a numbers game and the more men we can sift through, the more likely we are to find a good one, so online dating is just another potential way to meet more men.

But your chance of success here is dependent on your attitude; be positive.

4. Talk to men in real life

You might think there are no decent men out there. This belief often stems from the fact that the ones who approach you are the confident ones, the experienced ones, the ones with the moves. The nice guys that you could have a decent relationship with, they won't be so in-your-face, perhaps not so confident.

And you might think, 'I'm not interested in men who don't have the balls to approach me.' But there are a load of perfectly legitimate reasons why a good guy might keep away:

You look amazing – why would you be interested in him?

You're busy, he doesn't want to disturb you – he's considerate, remember.

He doesn't want to be that creep – he's respectful.

It's time to get off your phone, open your body posture, make eye contact and smile. And if he doesn't come and speak to you? There's nothing stopping you from speaking to him. It's the twenty-first century. Whatever you do, don't leave it up to the universe to deliver your man – it doesn't work like that. Make conversation, smile, put in some effort; make your own luck.

5. Get your self-esteem sorted

Finally, you need to know that you've got what it takes to be attractive to a man who's right for you. Everyone's different, so don't hide your uniqueness. If you've got a PhD in astrophysics and like doing maths in your spare time, some men will run a mile (they would never work anyway), but there will be someone out there who loves the idea of you and your quirks, and that is who you want. One woman I know wrote on her dating profile: 'Overeducated high-achiever with fantastic legs'. She met her current husband!

So put yourself out there and hold your head high. Good self-esteem and confidence, when you have them, are your most powerful tools. The self-esteem means you won't put up with bad behaviour, and the confidence will make you glow. And when you meet someone, instead of asking yourself, 'How can I be attractive to this guy?', it should be, 'Is this man showing up for me? Is he capable of being the kind of partner I need?' This is how to put yourself in the best position to find a fabulous relationship.

> *Secret: If you really want a new partner, think hard about what kind of man (if that is what you are after ...) you are attracted to. Are you falling into the evolutionary trap? Do you really need a tall, dark, rich player, or would a kinder, gentler kind of man who shares your values and interests actually be a better match? Maybe it's not that Mr Right isn't out there; it's just you are not seeing him.*

The courage it takes to love

When I set up Noon, my co-founder Claire (the real heroine of this book) sent me a card; it said: 'Do something that scares you every day!' Inside she had written: 'Only one?' I cherish that missive because although from the outside looking in, people think I am confident, the truth is often I am quaking inside but I power on through it. Often, I find the strength to persevere comes from the support of the people I love and who love me. I reckon it's important to say this because sometimes the stands we make that are most powerful are those which are the most frightening.

In that bracket I would definitely put speaking out on ITV news about the terrible comments made by British columnist and provocateur Jeremy Clarkson about Meghan Markle. He wrote that she should be pelted with excrement and paraded naked through the streets while crowds shouted 'Shame'. (He was referring to a scene from *Game of Thrones* but that didn't make it okay.) I couldn't understand why the *Sun*, a British tabloid newspaper, had published the column. I was Jeremy's editor for over ten years in my old life at the *Sunday Times*. Often, high-profile columnists, particularly those who are paid to be outrageous, step outside the line of what is publishable; the job of the editor is to know where the line is and to enforce it. We used to joke in the office about 'saving the big beasts from themselves'.

So when that column about Meghan ran I knew that it was either a massive mistake – no one senior enough had read it, though that was unlikely (and the paper eventually apologised) – or they had intentionally run it, knowing the distress it would cause. Either way, it wasn't okay. I knew that someone could have, and should have, either stopped it running altogether, or changed it to make it less misogynist, racist, inflammatory and offensive. I wanted the world to understand that perspective and process, so I set out to do the rounds of the TV studios, quaking with fear.

If you've been an insider and you then attack your old tribe it feels terrifying, whether that is justified or not. I tell this story because I want to stress how hard it is to go against everything you have been a part of, even when you know you are right and something really needs saying.

How much harder is it then, when, like Minna, everything you have been brought up to venerate, and have been part of, has to be rejected in order to save yourself. This is her amazingly brave account of how she not only left her Punjabi arranged marriage but then spoke out within her community against the stigma of divorce, to encourage other women not to suffer in silence. I love her story because it shows how, when we speak up with courage in spite of our fear, we act not just for ourselves and for what we need and know to be right, but for other women too. In our actions we light a torch of hope for others.

'As a midlife Punjabi woman, I am seen by most men within my community as being about as covetable as a scratched second-hand car. My crime? I am a Punjabi Sikh divorcee. Or a woman who was brave enough to leave her husband because she refused to accept a miserable emotional existence in order to still be considered "respectable". I realise that saying this out loud, even in 2024, may well confirm many of the outsider prejudices about the Punjabi community. That all our women are downtrodden, that there is something highly suspicious about how we can still rely upon "arranged" marriages to find life partners. But tragically some of those prejudices are still true, which is why I want other Punjabi women to hear my story and know they are not alone. That no one should be suffering in silence.'

Minna had always wanted a long and happy relationship like that of her parents, who came to the UK as first-generation immigrants in the 1960s and had an 'arranged' marriage the anglicised way – through a family friend and based only on a photo and scant information. Her family's life was woven into the spiritual fabric of the local gurdwara, or Sikh temple. They all volunteered there and Minna would often help the matrimonial team, a group within the temple set up to help observant men and women to meet and find love. They try to create matches through mutual compatibility; work, hobbies, biographies of families. It was through them that she was introduced to her now ex-husband.

'We were married shortly after we met. I was in my late twenties and feeling the pressure to get on with it. But within a year I realised he wasn't the guy I thought he was. I felt like I had suddenly stepped back in time. The relationship was very controlling and I was expected to kowtow to his mother and family at all times.'

She knew she had to get out. 'Luckily for me my parents were understanding, they didn't want me to be unhappy, so I returned home. In fact, I am still there.'

Minna feels wretched because as she gets older she is realising that she 'will have to choose between my faith, or finding someone I love because the available Punjabi men reject me, immediately, on the basis of my divorce. My appeal is tarnished, even among those who are also divorced. They want a younger, purer woman who can give them children. I would also like children, but have to battle the ageism that most 45-year-old women face. I feel like my community is riddled with these double standards, that Punjabi women struggle to have their voices heard. I know I am not the only one who chafes at how women are still seen to belong in the kitchen preparing the langar [food] while men are the Pardhan, or temple leaders.'

She explains that in her culture for a long time women have stayed quiet and accepted that the men are the leaders 'because we grew up seeing this played out and the women who came before us were too nervous to stand up for change. There is friction between younger women like me who want change and the older women who are scared of rocking the boat. This is obvious in the way the community reacted to my divorce. When I told some female friends my marriage was over, many turned their back on me, and the community I had felt safe in made me feel ashamed instead. I've been told to go to India to find a husband, but I know that if Punjabi men in London, who are already used to more independent women, are struggling to accept someone like me, it will never work with someone who is more traditional.'

This is a particular blow because Minna loves the temple and her faith. 'My choice to stand outside the expected behaviour of a Punjabi woman has been and continues to be tough. Frequently, I'm asked: "Have you met anyone?" When I say that it's hard to meet a decent guy who doesn't judge me, everyone thinks there is something wrong with me. I should be in the prime of my life, not feeling ashamed of my place in the world. I want to continue building my career and making a difference. Is it too much to expect that I would meet someone who is going to add value and light to my life? A man who is intelligent and understands that British Punjabi men and women can be equal?'

Not content just to stand by, Minna bravely established a weekly panel for Punjabi women called the Inspirational Women series, giving other women the opportunity to share their stories of standing up for change. 'It was frowned upon at first but it is now gathering momentum. I want other Punjabi women to know that we are all special regardless of our marital status. I was one of the first of any Punjabi women I knew who got divorced, and I remember that feeling of being alone and not having anyone to talk to. I felt permanently worried about what to say and was ashamed. But now I openly talk about my story; it is not shameful to be in your forties and divorced. Just because I am getting older does not mean my life is over, whatever the traditionalists might say. I can now see many women starting to stand up with me.

Inequalities will always exist but I am not going to sit back and stay silent.' Minna hopes that by speaking out she can help the women who come after her. 'We must not be shamed and silenced or afraid of labels and judgement. If things are going to change, we must be strong and brave. Society will always make us feel a certain way, but I want to say: Ignore the noise, my Punjabi sisters, and power up. What matters is that you, along with all midlife women, know that you are amazing and beautiful and can achieve anything you want. You just have to believe you can.'

Indeed.

One of the great joys of my work with women in midlife is meeting women from different worlds and backgrounds – like Minna. There is some terrifying research in America which shows that most corporate professionals have *no* black or Asian friends, or none who are close enough to come round to their house for dinner.

That is a shame because I have found that the friendships I have formed with BAME women have done more to challenge and enrich my life and viewpoints than almost anything else. At a recent Noon retreat I was standing chatting to two black female friends. They were talking about how there is no equivalent in white culture to being called 'Auntie': Lesley was saying she'd popped into the hairdresser's in Brixton to get her braids redone and the young woman had gone: 'Here's your chair, Auntie!' Lesley explained that 'Auntie' was a term of respect accorded to an older woman in her Caribbean community, one who had earnt her stripes – but it in no way meant that woman was sexually past it or old. It was more of a tip of the hat to that woman's wonderful, vintage fabulousness. A celebration of her Queenly qualities.

The closest I could think of was when I go into my local Italian deli and they call me 'Signora', or if you go to France and they call you 'Madame' not 'Mademoiselle'. But I don't think that is quite the same as both of those are about a woman's marital status, being Mrs not Miss. Whereas 'Auntie' packs a celebratory punch about being a respected older woman. I've witnessed this in Jamaica, too. I was playing pickleball with a group of Queenagers out there. Next to us were about twenty local youths all playing football. Their goal was right next to our court. 'Could you lot play at the other end of the pitch?' one local older lady asked. Immediately, the boys stopped kicking the ball at us and did what she asked. Now, I just can't imagine that ever happening in London. In Jamaica an older woman is treated with respect, obeyed instantly. In the West? Not so much … In fact, if I asked a group of young men in London to relocate their game I would expect either to be ignored or ridiculed. Which is, I suppose, at the heart of what this book is about – changing the story and the value that our culture puts on older women.

One of the women who has radically challenged my views on everything from veils to the Islamic practice of taking more than one wife is my friend Fatima. We met years ago on a panel about female leadership and spent an afternoon hanging out together in our hotel. We've been chatting ever since. Fatima comes from a town in the north of England which is a byword for racial tensions; where in one of the first waves of immigration thousands of Pakistani men came to work in the cotton mills, which subsequently went bust.

Unusually in her community, Fatima is nearly fifty, a successful businesswoman who makes deals all around the world in the 'halal' economy (the Muslim market is worth trillions!) and who happens to be single and childfree. She wears a hijab, and is quietly, and profoundly, devout. One of the first conversations we had was about her decision to wear hijab. I, like many Western women, had always seen the veil as a symbol of female oppression. But Fatima explained that was not the case at all, that she had started wearing hijab (a headscarf which covers the hair and wraps around the neck, along with modest dress that reaches to the ground) in her teens as an act of rebellion. 'My parents hated it; they didn't want me to look so "different", they were all about fitting into Britain and looking more secular outside the home. It didn't go down well with school either, they thought it was repressive. So that was a win for me, it annoyed my parents and my teachers! Result!'

Fatima explains that wearing hijab gave her a sense of power and agency. 'Women like me who wear it have choices. It means no one has an automatic right to see me or touch me. I choose who shakes my hand, who hugs me, or kisses me; strangers can't touch me or see me. Only those whom I choose can see my full face, or my hair or the contours of my body. I like that I am not always on display, that there is no pressure to look perfect. I am an undiscovered continent. Hijab sends the message: I have boundaries. Respect me. Respect my boundaries.' She feels hijab gives her power over her sexuality and when she unleashes it.

That doesn't mean Fatima doesn't get offers from men. Quite the contrary. I found the Muslim way of courtship fascinating. 'I think of my suitors like jam jars – I've currently got ten who are interested, at least half of whom want to marry me. I was in Turkey the other day and an older businessman said very seriously to me that he wanted to be my husband. I said, "Get in the queue, there are about eight in front of you." He said: "Seriously, put me in at number nine!" I have had at least thirty marriage proposals but I am ferociously independent. I like to run my own life. I decided that small children would be incompatible with my life path; I like to work. I didn't want my own family; I have lots of nieces and nephews in my extended family whom I love dearly.'

Fatima had an unhappy arranged marriage when she was twenty to a man who had just arrived from Pakistan and found her too opinion-ated, too educated (she was the first person in her family to go to university, and got a master's degree from Oxford). She had to battle to get out of the marriage and was helped by her father, 'who could see my husband wasn't good enough for me'. It took about eight years to finally extricate herself and, like Minna, she was stigmatised in her community, although she says that many of the men who did that have since apologised. 'I was just ahead of the curve because these days about a third of the women I know have been divorced. I suppose that, because we have our children so young – in our early twenties – by the time the women are in their late thirties or forties they are free of family ties, they go travelling, start businesses, go back to study, do their own thing. Remarry for love, someone they chose. There are many independent women in my community.'

We talked about the Muslim practice whereby men can take more than one wife. 'It is not what you think. In our culture the first wife might be an arranged marriage, she will be the mother of his children. Then later he might fall in love. But rather than leaving his first wife and the family and the children as is common in wider British culture, many men stay and support the original wife; she retains her status and her home, but he also has a second wife which is his love match.' Fatima says she has considered becoming a second wife herself but has always decided against it in the end because she cherishes her independence.

She explains that neither hijab nor her religion prohibit dating or relationships. 'I have lots of suitors, I am a fan of WhatsApp because it is encrypted; we meet for coffee and things. There is even some-thing called a "Muta", which is a time-limited version of the "Nikkah", the simple religious pledge made in front of God which is the key component of marriage. A Muta means that in the eyes of God you can be "married" for twenty-four hours or a week so that you can try out a new relationship.' Although as ever a double standard operates. 'Men can look down on you for doing a Muta, but it does mean that relationships are possible.'

Marriages in her British Pakistani community, she explains, are often arranged to further family businesses, or for social-climbing reasons. 'When my community first came to the UK they would club together to afford a house, and all live in it together to save money for the next one, until everyone had a house – without having to go near a bank. That system can work very well: if you live in a multi-generational household and you go out to work, there is someone to look after the children, to do the cooking, everyone mucks in to clean. The downside is that everybody knows your business, there isn't much privacy.'

Fatima is particularly interested in my work around midlife because in her world Queenagers don't feel powerless and invisible. 'Older women rule everything in my culture! The mum in the household is the Queen, she is on a throne, she controls the daughters-in-law, who live with her, the finances (she has the gold), her husband … If there is abuse in our families these powerful older women are often the perpetrators. They rule with an iron rod. This issue, with women over fifty feeling invisible, is a Western construct, because in that culture women are encouraged to perform in every aspect of their lives and are constantly compared sexually and physically to younger women. That does not happen in our culture. Each kind of women has her place and a different power. Queenagers are valued and are naturally in synergy in the Islamic world and in the global south.'

It's like that in business in her community too. 'I notice white entrepreneurs venerate youth, but I am always looking for grey hair, for wisdom; older people can have energy and vibrancy too, but they also have experience.'

What Fatima does find is that she is constantly underestimated. 'I was brought up by my father who adored me to be tough; to fight back. I am brilliant at putting together deals and I will not be undercut. I stand my ground and say, "Why are you disrespecting me?" That usually terrifies them!'

Secret: Make friends with a Queenager or two who are different from you – learn about the world and relationships from their point of view and don't make assumptions that your way is the only way, or that all cultures are dismissive of older women.

Friends – the greatest love of all

The sun was shining and the white plumage of a gull caught my eye as I walked to the steps of the pond. The water was chilly on my ankles, colder over the knees. In winter, when the pond is only 7 degrees, immersion has to be slow and conscious. As the cold rises up and up, over my waist and chest, I have learnt to breathe out slowly, forcing the body to be calm. Overriding the reflex to flee, panic, not get into the freezing water.

I can tell the swimmers who aren't used to it. They plunge into the water whooping and squealing, gasping at the cold. Us regulars know to exhale as we submerge into the chill. The first few strokes are the most intense, the cold seems to cut, but then the brain adjusts, breathing regulates and the world becomes sparkly. There is only *now*.

Green parakeets screech over the trees. I swim in a straight line into the sun, close my eyes – within and without is dazzling light. To my left the sun illuminates the leafless branches, burnishing stems gold and red in the wintry light. I love the minutiae of small difference; returning to the same spot almost every day it is always the same, but also always not. The willow fronds will have greened since the day before, or buds begun to swell. Some days gulls cry and swoop. Or the surface of the water ripples, ruffled by wind. Other times it is still, glassy – polished pewter, skeleton branches reflected so they seem both above and below. I watch for magpies, reading the runes: one for sorrow, two for joy. Chiding myself for being superstitious.

Or I notice tiny blue tits fluttering high in the naked branches, always together.

Those small changes, noticing them; that is evidence of life.

Nowhere is that clearer than in the people we love. As I swam that day I smiled to myself. The evening before, I'd had dinner with one of my oldest friends. We have known each other for more than thirty years. There's that old truism about friends being for a season, for a reason, or forever. She is one of those rare birds in the third bracket.

If I'm sad I know I can pick up the phone and even if I am crying so hard I can't speak – something that's happened quite a lot in the last three years – she will be there on the end of the line, her voice soft: 'What's wrong, Elsy, what is it?' On days where the words are muffled by snot and sadness she'll listen to me snuffling and heaving until I can speak; and it will then all be all right. I will be heard. It will be okay to be sad. I've learnt how important it is to let the shutters up on the misery, to let someone in. Not keep the game face on with the ones who love you – because there is *nothing* lonelier than that. For me the true measure of love, of connection and acceptance, is being able to speak with no filter, no fear of judgement – knowing that the other person understands. Being able to speak from one soul to another in pure communication. That has to be at the heart of all of our most intimate relationships. Otherwise what are they for?

But I have also learnt that that quality of intimacy can expand and contract. That everyone copes with grief differently. It is only now my friend has come back to life that I realise how sad she has been for a while; how frozen, how stuck. She moved far away. I thought the distance between us was just that. Distance. We were both at full stretch, juggling jobs and kids. I saw her infrequently and when I did she seemed stressed. But it's hard in a café over coffee with phones bleeping and kids interrupting to see a friend clearly. Same at dinner with other friends, or even when it was just us. She seemed constantly distracted, frenetic, aloof, impossible to pin down.

We've always laughed together. No – we've done more than laughed; we've pratted about, made up daft nicknames, and dances; giggled at stupid things, travelled the world, spent hours on Rightmove imagining new futures closer together. But for a while, I thought that person had gone. The lights were off. She seemed cold. Shut off. After some of our meetings I almost wondered if we were still friends.

And then I went to stay and discovered what she wasn't telling me; that she and her partner were living in parallel worlds. That if he came into a room, she would walk out of it. There was no casual touching, no shared jokes, just curt orders. It felt uncomfortable to be around them. When we went to the big bedroom so she could show me her new leather jacket, I noticed his clothes were gone from the wardrobe.

He seemed to be sleeping in the study/summerhouse at the bottom of the garden, despite the chill; not just emotional but physical, it was winter, snow on the ground. At meals, everyone raided the fridge and took their food off to a different room. The eldest boy in the kitchen, the husband in his shed. Me and my friend on the patio (in February).

The old communality of the family, the sharing, the jokes, were absent. There was no centre, no heart. I remember another friend saying shortly before her own divorce that her marriage was like one of those old-fashioned spinning wheels on a cart – all iron struts and a void at the centre of the circle where the love should be.

That week we went on long, cold walks with a hyperactive dog. My friend was walking so fast I had to jog to keep up. Noting my laboured breathing, she said usually she ran this route, up and down hills, through woods, twice a day. I wanted to ask what she was running away from. But I didn't.

It is hard to know what to do when a friend is unhappy. My emotions run close to the surface, I find them hard to contain, it all spills out. Others deal with sadness not with outbursts of snot and sniffing, but stoicism. When they don't share, it is hard to ask. I've learnt that you just have to wait till they are ready. For the thaw.

Late one night she cracked. 'I'm going to leave him,' she said, as the credits rolled on *Working Girl*, one of our old favourite films. 'I just haven't told him yet … I'm worried about the kids.'

I nodded. She gave me a swift peck on the cheek and disappeared up to her lonely ex-marital bed. I sat in her lounge, looking at the pictures of happier times. The wedding – the two of them entwined, giddy with hope. Her with her eldest, hands held tight. The four of them on a blustery beach, bright smiles defying the wind. I felt what she had no words to say. The end of what had been good. The hundreds of days of frostiness and contempt. The way her intimate witness had become a stranger.

The next few months were tough.

A text: 'I've told him. We're talking to lawyers. Nightmare.' A late-night call. Concern about her youngest son. 'He's acting up at school. Was caught with dope. He says he's depressed. I'm a terrible mother.' That overpowering feeling of uselessness on the end of a phone. 'It will be okay,' I said. 'Kids are more resilient than you think. All 14-year-olds have a shit time. He's a good kid.' I could hear the fear, the guilt, the worry in her voice.

Then the actual split.

This is my new number. My new address. A weekend when she came to stay. Her concern about her teenagers. But also a tremulous giggle after a couple of glasses of wine. Her girlishly showing me her new online dating profile.

She moved back near me. Our meetings became more regular again. Joy. She had a new haircut. A natty new leather jacket; bright-hued this time. A snazzy white jumpsuit. I teased. She giggled. Then a confession. 'I've met someone!' She'd found him online. He was widowed, and had two older kids. They'd been on three dates. She was wondering whether to have him to stay. The kids were with their dad that weekend. (He had also found a new partner.) It was like we were teenagers again. She confessed that the new man was a good snog, and laughed. We joked about how long it was since she'd had sex. Would she be able to do it? Was she a born-again virgin? She confessed it had been years. I hugged her tight, wishing I'd known. She shook her head. 'I couldn't say,' she said. 'It felt so disloyal to him. You know him too.' I thought about the things that don't get said, even between the oldest of friends.

The date turned out to be a frog. But she persisted with the online app. A few months later we were out for a weekend walk, laughing at the dog sniffing endless bottoms.

I realised we were back to where we'd always been. That she was back. I looked at her closely. She smiled with her eyes again. I was glad.

Sometimes in the relationships we cherish most, those which embody the biggest loves we have in our lives, we have to learn to wait. To accept that if we are patient and loving, the deep freeze will be followed by a thaw. There will be spring again. Some things can't be forced; they have their own rhythm. In these relationships, we need to be alive to the minutiae of small differences and not give up.

In my life I've learnt that love comes in many forms, that it can arrive when we least expect it to. The big love of my life walked up some steps and found me when I was reading a book. One minute he didn't exist, the next he was there, and three decades later he has never left.

I have also come to learn that love requires us to be brave; remember the old adage: caution in love is the worst form of caution. When it comes to love no one can do it for us; we have to make the leap into vulnerability all by ourselves – open up our tender, fragile hearts to the possibility of true connection. Let ourselves be truly seen in all our grandeur and brokenness. Because in that leap of trust, miracles happen.

Secret: Love – in all its forms, whether romantic or between friends – is always worth the risk, worth the effort, worth the wait. It is the sparkle, the joy that makes everything in life worthwhile.

PART THREE

FAMILY

Do you have kids? It's one of those questions that women get asked all the time, which, if we stop and think about it, is both incredibly personal and rudely intrusive. It sounds so innocuous, but in the answer can lie a lifetime of unrequited longing, tragedy, or indeed an understandable sense that a woman does not need kids to complete her.

It used to be that by fifty that mother question was moot; the conversation became menopause not maternity. But not anymore. I went to a party and bumped into a friend who was two years ahead of me at uni. 'Is the primary school at the end of your road any good?' she asked. Turns out she has a 4-year-old daughter! It's a peculiar facet of our Queenager generation that at fifty you can, like me, have an 18- and 21-year-old, or grandchildren, or kids at primary school, or a 4-year-old – or for nearly a third of us (and the more educated we are, the fewer sprogs we have) no kids at all. Which is quite a leveller!

I am very careful at our Noon Circles never to assume that all Queenagers are mothers. The whole point of this book is to challenge the fecund/fuckable patriarchal view of women (i.e. that we only have value from the male perspective if we are fertile and could have kids and/or we are fanciable). Part of changing the narrative about how we see women in midlife and beyond is thinking about what women are for, what they can do and the legacy they leave, in a new way – not thinking that whether we are mothers or not is all-defining. Women have so many wonderful qualities which improve with age – wisdom, experience, creativity, kindness. These days, children are not our only possible legacy; just because we have a womb doesn't mean we have to procreate! Nearly half of our childfree Queenagers at Noon have actively chosen *not* to be mothers. Good for them. Many are at pains to point out, though, that just because they aren't mums doesn't mean they don't have kids in their life whom they love and are close to. I love their tales of being wonderful aunties, godmothers or step-parents (never easy, but not all stepmothers are monsters – I loved mine!).

That said, for many of us our biggest midlife challenges stem from our children. Whether that's the knackeration of having them when we are older and just surviving the sleep deprivation, or the challenge of our Gen Z teens grappling with an epidemic of mental health issues. Coping with that is one of the hardest things any of us will ever have to face. I hope that the very honest account in this section of dealing with an anorexic teen will help readers empathise with anyone they know who is in a similar situation.

If we survive the teen years we are then rewarded with the grief of losing our hands-on parenting role when the little darlings fly the nest. It is so strange to go from caring for children every day to them being out and off in the big wide world. Suddenly feeling redundant as a mother, in terms of the day-to-day, unexpectedly floored me. The empty nest is another way that Queenagers are forced to pivot into a new phase.

So, whether we have them or not, children are a big part of midlife and our becoming. This is what we will be exploring in this section.

Do you have kids?

It is increasingly common for Queenagers of my generation not to have children; nearly 30 per cent of women who went on to higher education don't have kids, according to the latest UK statistics, and the more successful a woman is in terms of a career, the more likely she is not to have them. This is also true in the US, where the missing children of career women have been written about in books such as *Baby Hunger* by Sylvia Ann Hewlett. Indeed, globally, the more highly educated a woman is, the less likely she is to have kids. (This is not true of men.) I see this very clearly in my own friendship circle; around a third of my female peers from Oxford University are childfree.

When we were younger and some of us started becoming mothers and some didn't, it created tension and separation. I'm guilty of that too. When my kids were small, I was so exhausted by trying to navigate holding down a big job and caring for my little ones that there was no room for friends or socialising. Many friendships fell away. Having had some long and honest conversations with women about this since, I realise my own self-absorption (you could call this survival mode!) was unintentionally hurtful.

My great pal Karen, who couldn't have children due to early menopause, put it to me like this:

'It's like a double grief, your own because kids might have been something you've longed for and then can't have. Plus the sadness of losing connection with your dearest friends as they enter a world of which you are not a part. I found I had nothing to say in conversations about weaning, or nappies, or which schools to choose. And those end-of-the-day phone calls I used to share with my girlfriends, when we used to just catch up and chat amicably about our lives, also ceased as the mothers disappeared into a new whirlwind of parenthood. It was doubly hard. To feel rejected and excluded and to want what they had – and to be dealing with my own grief about what was not to be.'

Karen says she found some peace by holding a ceremony – like a memorial, or a marking – for the loss of the children she'd never had.

'I compare it in a way to losing a child. Everyone is sympathetic about that; to lose a child is one of the cruellest blows. But if, like me, you couldn't have children because of your own body not being able to be pregnant, then there is a huge grief, like a bereavement, for those children you desperately wanted, but didn't have. But unlike a child that lives and dies there is no public way of marking that, of mourning for it, for this massive, painful absence. For me, the closure provided by that ritual, my ceremony, was incredibly healing.'

Like many childfree women, Karen is very close to her nieces and nephews and is a much-loved godmother; she has intentionally channelled her latent maternal energy into her legacy project. 'My work now is about supporting the leaders of the future, nurturing a new generation in a different way. I find many childfree women want to create a different kind of legacy which connects us to the future. To channel our nurturing and creative natures in new ways. To create new models of what our lives can be, what they can look like. But it is not talked about or recognised more widely, which is also hard.'

The stories of childfree women, whether that was their intention or just what they were dealt, are rarely told in our culture; these women are often made to feel less than, or odd, when that choice is increasingly mainstream. It is an area we have leant into at Noon because many of them feel irritated to be so unseen, when their situation is so common. I find it incomprehensible that more brands – particularly those flogging luxury items or financial products – don't actively target the childfree. As one woman – a partner in a London law firm, who is fifty and has no kids – put it to me: 'I am disposable-income-erama. I have a fat salary and no kids, yet no brands target me … it's crazy.' I'm afraid the reason for this omission is the male lens, which too often governs the way the media and thus our culture portrays women. It's a viewpoint that doesn't value a childfree woman and, lazily, no one bothers to challenge the outdated stereotype, even though the childfree make up a whopping third of the Queenager cohort and are likely to be the wealthiest.

This aspect of Queenager life is most in need of a new lens. That is why I am so proud to tell Kerensa Jennings' story. Kerensa gave herself a 'magic permission pass' to live her life on her own terms. She likens it to an imaginary 'get out of jail free' card, a way of telling herself: Permission granted. You are officially allowed not to have children and to carve out your life the way you want.

She explained that this is so necessary because when women deviate from convention they inevitably 'tread gingerly, wondering if we've made a big mistake'. Kerensa says that, 'Deciding early on in life that I didn't want to be a mother was one of those mega moments in my life. For ages I felt I was being judged. One senior (male) executive I worked with asked if there was "something wrong with my bits". This was just one of countless tasteless comments which I've found hurtful and unkind. Just as pregnant friends complain about strangers stroking their bulging bellies, it's unsettling when people think it's okay to invade your space with opinions about your childlessness. It's none of their business.'

She says she finds herself being 'defensive' every time the question is asked. 'I always feel the need to explain that it was my choice not to be a mother and that I have wonderful children in my life – my two nieces, my nephew, my goddaughter and my godson, and, since my marriage, two stepdaughters. I want people to think I am normal, not weird, so I find myself justifying the absence of a child in my home, or an empty nest, by reassuring my interrogator that I *love* children so they don't think I'm an alpha cyborg, devoid of emotion and tenderness.'

Kerensa also dreads what she calls 'that powerful, beautiful, but also alienating phrase "as a mother…".' It makes her cry inside.

It is really important that the choices and stories of women like Kerensa are more widely understood. She explained her decision was partly due to a family tragedy; her parents had a premature son who died within days the year before she was born. Her mother never got to hold him and he has no grave. She was incredulous when she finally heard the story and felt 'unbelievably sad and a bit betrayed. I couldn't believe I hadn't been told something so fundamental.' It turned out her mother had had several miscarriages and had been hospitalised for much of her pregnancy with Kerensa.

'Rewinding the story of how many years of suffering Mum had experienced was behind me making up my mind by the time I was fifteen that I would never have children – particularly since I had to have part of my cervix removed when a smear test discovered pre-cancerous cells. Plus, I had a premature menopause in my thirties and remember feeling thankful that I had already taken the life-defining decision about not having children of my own.'

As a childfree woman at work, Kerensa has also felt an 'expectation from colleagues that my own plans should be sacrificed for their nativity plays, sports days or looking after a child with chickenpox. I mostly haven't minded, because of course I understand. And in fact, a lot of the time, those things *are* more important than whatever I had going on. But there has been the odd occasion when I have had to give up something that mattered a lot to me – and I'm not sure it was ever appreciated.'

In my own experience of being a boss, I know how often those without kids have had to pick up the strain over half term or Christmas. With the benefit of hindsight, I would do things differently. We all need to remember that those without children have personal commitments that matter too. They also have people to take care of – we may not all be parents but we all have parents who will age and need looking after – and we all have projects that are important to us. Talking to Kerensa made me think about whether I could have been more understanding around that issue, and it also made me realise the immense 'soul nourishment', as she puts it, that she and others like her have found in their work. Kerensa has been part of creating TV shows with everyone from Nelson Mandela to Sir David Attenborough – on everything from palaeontology to politics. She's travelled the globe for work and is particularly proud of her (wonderful) novel *Seas of Snow*, which she sees as 'my baby. My own mum jokes it had a much longer gestation than most babies, and she is right (seven years!).'

The creativity of childfree women like Kerensa is often channelled into different forms of legacy, whether that is a novel, or a charity, or a cause. 'I also have a cat I adore, and although I have had a bumpy road in matters of the heart, I do feel somewhat late in life that I have at last landed in a place where I love, and am loved. At no point, though, have I ever felt an empty hollow where a child should be. In my own life, I made the right decision.'

That is not to say that she hasn't had her share of tough times. Like all of us, she has. But I like her remedy for that: 'I get through life's tricky bits by running through my grateful list every day before I get out of bed, reminding myself of my blessings. I find that infuses my day with sunshine and positivity.' Like me, she has learnt to tap into her wellsprings of joy: 'I love writing and also little things – hearing rain, watching the zoo of butterflies, bees, robins, magpies, squirrels, turtle doves, herons and frogs that use my garden as a social club. I like quietness and to feel serene somewhere calm and beautiful. I am an introvert and am energised by being alone with my thoughts.'

Kerensa has created a life that suits her; a life that is, as Nancy put it to me that day on the boat, resonant. Her outside matching her inside.

I love the message that we can all find fulfilment in different ways, that we each need to forge our own path and have the 'confidence to be me'.

It has taken me fifty-two years to discover that it is absolutely fine to be me, just as I am. Try repeating that to yourself – 'I am enough, just as I am' – over and over if necessary until you believe it. Then you can write your own magic permission pass. Kerensa swears it is the 'best present you can give yourself. Do things your way. Be different. Follow your heart. Don't wait for someone else to give you permission. Or tell you you're "officially allowed". Believe me – you are.'

Secret: Give yourself a magic permission pass. It's your life – you choose what suits you and how you want to live it! Learn to ask for forgiveness, not permission. That really is a game changer!

Having kids 'late' in life

We Queenagers are pioneers; there has never been a cohort of women like us before who have worked from graduation, through maternity and hung in there. In the 2019 UK census women over forty started outearning women under forty for the first time *ever*. And one of the consequences of that is financially assisted later motherhood. Some Queenagers now have resources and choices that earlier women didn't have – I'm talking about using sperm donors, egg donors and even surrogates to start a family when the natural fertility window has closed. This is a choice that was not open to earlier generations. And while the 50-year-old mum club is small, it is also high profile, with celebrities such as Naomi Campbell, Natalie Massenet (founder of NET-A-PORTER) and Sarah Jessica Parker leading the way.

It's not just celebrities. A growing number of solvent, professional women are choosing to go it alone as mothers in their mid-forties, fifties and beyond. The first woman I knew personally who became a late mum on her own was a work colleague. She was senior, super-competent, romantically challenged – in that she couldn't find someone she wanted to settle down with – and had always wanted to be a mother. In her late forties she did IVF with donor sperm and got pregnant. I bumped into her at the pond – I was showering naked, while she waxed lyrical about her son, 'the best thing I ever did'.

I went on a walk with another late-life mum, Denise. She'd devoted her thirties and forties to her career; then, in her fifties, she decided she wanted to have kids. Like an increasing number of older successful women, Denise is upending the usual pattern of life. I had kids in my early thirties and, with the support of my husband, who was incredibly hands-on, I somehow struggled through being an editor and a mum. Denise did the opposite. She told me how, despite having built a successful career, she still felt a void, an emptiness in her life which she felt just couldn't be filled by her financial and professional success. She couldn't help but look around at her male contemporaries, who were marrying younger women, or on their second wife, and see how they were enjoying all the upsides of corporate success *and* a rich family hinterland as well. Denise had always longed to be a mother and knew she would be a good one, so she spent a fortune on IVF, donor eggs and sperm, and was one of the lucky ones. When I remarked that it must be quite a load, being a single corporate mum, she laughed and explained that she has a full-time nanny who lives down the hall, and because she doesn't have a romantic relationship to manage too, she can log back on to work after the kids are in bed. She reckoned she had the best of both worlds. She felt that in some ways she had struck a blow for feminism: men have been having kids later forever, so why shouldn't women? To her, that was true equality.

But what does it really take to become a mother, alone, in your fifties? Linnet is a banker who lives in the Middle East. She was in her early forties when she first started thinking about having children without a man. Her reasoning was that 'if I died without ever having been married that wouldn't be so bad. But if I died without ever having had children, that was just simply too devastating to even think about. So I began researching freezing my eggs and finally did it when I was forty-five.' She harvested sixteen eggs and thought that since she only wanted two children, all would be well, so she upped sticks and followed her career abroad. Once in the Middle East, life was a whirl of horse riding, socialising and ballroom dancing. But her desire for children did not disappear.

'The complication for me was that I wanted any child of mine to have a father, even if not in the traditional family sense. And since my life had firmly transitioned to my new homeland, that meant someone living in the same country as me. Five years later this person appeared, a good male friend, someone who also wanted a child and who had a positive attitude towards a co-parenting arrangement. We jumped through all the complex co-parenting arrangement hoops (lots of counselling and paperwork, primarily) and we used his sperm to fertilise my frozen eggs in London. From my sixteen eggs, a few embryos developed but the pre-genetic testing revealed that they were all too deficient and not worth transferring.' It was a horribly harsh and unexpected blow. Linnet was determined not to give up and two months later went to an IVF clinic in South America, where embryos created with donor eggs and her friend's sperm were implanted.

The IVF was successful and eight months later her son arrived. She and her co-parent moved to live close together and when she returned to work they shared custody 50:50. 'The only problem was, I really missed having a child at home when my son went to stay with his father, so I decided to have more children. In fact, I really wanted to have twins so that they would always have each other. My friend didn't want to have any more children so this time I went it alone using donor eggs and an anonymous sperm donor.'

It took three attempts this time, but it was worth the wait. 'I already had my son and now, at fifty-four years old, I had also become the proud mother of twins, a girl and a boy. I am now fifty-seven, and have just had a fourth child, another little boy. The clinic were amazed! Life is full and busy.'

Linnet has no regrets. Sure, she can't remember the last time she bought new shoes or a handbag, and she doesn't ride horses anymore. But when I ask her if it has all been worth it, she says: 'Absolutely, resoundingly, yes. Having waited so long to have children I had already done all the other things that I wanted to do. And my financial position is sufficient to provide as necessary, especially when it comes to the help I can afford to ensure that I can both work and rest as required. The children are now by far the most fun part of my life. I finally feel complete.'

Successful older men have often had children later in life with a younger partner. With the help of technology this door is now open to some women too. Hooray for the Queenager mothers. I salute their stamina. The broken nights nearly killed me when I was thirty; I am sure I couldn't do it now, but if Queenager-hood is all about fulfilling our dreams and motherhood is one of them – then why not?

Secret: Modern times and technology mean that if we have the resources we can create our own timelines when it comes to kids … never say never.

The teenage years

The blossom is frothing: armies of horse chestnuts proudly holding white candles aloft, cow parsley in full show, a three-dimensional technicolour feast of rhododendrons and, of course, the glorious, eponymous May flower. In terms of nature, it's my favourite time of year – like Gaia is just shrieking at us to notice her, appreciate her, feel grateful for the limitless abundance of spring celebrating life itself.

And yet this is a time of paradox. It is also exam time, stress time and, I suppose fittingly, it is Mental Health Month. I chaired a panel where an outwardly highly successful young man shared his own story of how his big tech job was derailed by a panic attack so bad he thought he was dying and was taken to hospital with what he assumed was a heart attack. It turned out to be a decade of suppressed feelings. He talked so fluently and beautifully about how he healed himself finally by tuning in to his emotions, not ignoring them – by asking for help, by practising everything from cold water immersion to breath work to yoga and meditation, so that when the anxiety strikes he has tools to tackle it. But also he talked about how 60 per cent of the workforce feels anxious to some degree, with women and Gen Z (our kids) the most affected.

That resonated with me because my youngest was mid-A levels. We have now parented through two sets of GCSEs and A levels as a family (one lot concurrent); I'm used to the house being full of revising teens who emerge every few hours to make more tea and smoke 'blems' (cigarettes) on our balcony. I spend hours lying on my daughter's bed while she makes politics essay plans. I listen to podcasts and read a book; she just likes me to be there. I squeeze her foot occasionally, go out and buy Oreos, bring up cups of tea, agree that revision is the pits, say encouraging things about how this is the gateway to a summer of fun and a new life at uni.

I've learnt over the years that the most useful thing I can do when my girls are anxious or stressed is to be a comforting presence, just there with sustenance and reassurance. They hate it if I grill them about whether they are doing enough, or about exam specifics; they torture and pressurise themselves too much anyway. The best way to help is to ask what they need in that moment and show up with it, whether that's a cup of tea, or popping out to buy sweets, or a hug, or running a bath. It's hard not to lecture, or interfere – or project our own anxieties about the whole of their future (gulp) into the mix. But our job here is to keep them as calm as possible; to suggest by our behaviour that we know they've got this. Not pile on extra stress. Some parents might find it weird that I allow a bit of a revision party to be going on – but everyone is different. My little one is naturally affiliative; she's always hated being alone. She takes comfort from what her peers call 'doubling' – just having someone around. She says it relaxes her to know someone is with her as she revises.

Not all kids are the same. The boys seem to work in a frantic, frenzied, head-down final sprint. One mate's son goes to the gym at 6.30am and by 8am is at the table swotting. Others have sons in meltdown. One Queenager who thought her straight-A son had his exam prep under control discovered he hadn't slept for a week and was hallucinating with anxiety and terror. Another was in hospital last week with her daughter who is dyslexic with severe ADHD and who began hearing voices and needed professional help. This is way more common than we might think; a third of Queenagers report their teens have mental illness, whether it's anxiety or anorexia, ADHD or self-harm. The Gen Z mental health crisis is real.

At such times all we can do as parents is be there, show up. Put down the other things going on in our lives to just be present. It's like going back to parenting a newborn baby or a toddler because much of what is required is pre-verbal; they need constant reassurance, and regular feeding, and sometimes you just have to lie with them and sing to them like you would a baby to get them to go to sleep. These are the most worrying times; as mothers we have to dig deep, call up all our reserves of self-control and sympathy; put aside our own feelings and concerns and just be there for them. The aim, a therapist told me, is to be like a Saint Bernard dog. Walking alongside, nudging them back in the right direction, providing tea or hot milk when required. There. Faithful. Dogged. A solid point, like the bottom of the swimming pool for them to push against and return to the light.

We live in a time when anxiety has reached epidemic proportions among our teens and young people. Parents now have to cultivate these soft skills, of being alongside, of containing, of being a quiet, faithful presence. To think about what our children need from us, not what we want/expect from them. This is a time when our own needs are truly secondary. Of course you will be feeling guilty, and emotional and triggered, so go and get some help, from a friend or, even better, a therapist. Your child can't handle your anxiety too. This is a time when, however bad you feel, you need to be contained for them; show them only your best, calm self. There is nothing like having a stressed/ill teen to make you realise as a parent that all your ambitions for them are meaningless compared to them just being happy. That nothing matters at all when they are really in the doldrums except keeping them alive, getting them through, seeing them smile again. That that really is everything.

I write this because I know how many kids – and therefore by extension parents – are in this zone during exam time and generally. The truth is that parenting teens is less intensive than having small kids; but when teens need you, they need *you* and no one else will do.

Anyone kind and loving can feed gloop to your baby, or cuddle your toddler. Small children, small problems. But when it comes to big children, think big problems! Sometimes it can feel like teenagers have regressed to toddler-dom – they need us there for a while to make the world all right again.

Given how many of us are grappling with teens with anxiety, often expressed through self-harm or eating disorders, I share this account from a therapist in Chicago whose daughter developed anorexia. If that is where you are now, I send you love and sympathy – your young person will get better. And if you are a childfree Queenager with a friend in this situation, wow, she needs you now.

When I spoke to Emma about her teenage daughter with anorexia it was hard to tally the composed professional therapist who appeared on my screen with the chaos she described unfolding at home. But it is that very need to keep up appearances for external life to carry on which takes such a toll. She explained how every day she or her husband had to get up at 6.45 to have their daughter's breakfast ready at 7.20. That morning she had been woken at 8am by the sobbing, choking and growling of her daughter 'losing her shit' over eating a spoonful of apple with her bran flakes. 'I immediately had this sense of huge doom descending as I could hear the wails that we now call the "Mewing Dragon" emanating from the kitchen. It's our personal code for her at her worst, when she becomes a terrorising horror.'

She explained that what helps her is to imagine her daughter has a wolf howling in her mind which attacks her if Emma or her Dad puts too much yoghurt on her porridge. 'The reasons for the anxious freakouts are so paltry, they curdle my heart in resentment and hate. But her distress is all too real. It makes her scream, head-bang walls, scrape the flesh off her calves with her nails. These violent moments of psychotic intensity are just part of daily family life now. Some days we negotiate her dinner of sweet potato, spinach and lentils without incident, but only if I have served *exactly* two spoons of sweet potato, not a speck more, and have chatted to her throughout about her school day, basketball match, etc.'

While this performance goes on, Emma's two younger sons sit in silence watching anxiously. 'She is a tyrant. The whole family sits there battle-ready. I can't pay attention to the other children during dinner time because she monopolises my attention entirely, then after dinner we must play cards or watch a movie (so she can't make herself sick). My attention must not wane. No matter that on some weekdays I have seen nine patients back-to-back since 8 in the morning, gone to her school on the northside by Lake Michigan with lunch and sat with her while she eats it. This is high-wire stuff. There are no breaks. Any lapse on my side and she panics. Her breaths come so fast I worry she will suffocate.'

Emma's natural maternal concern is mixed with equally natural extreme irritation. 'Sometimes I have to go out into my car and scream "HATE, HATE, HATE!" at the top of my voice to release some of my anger. I know it sounds mad but it helps.'

The toll on the wider family and Emma and her husband is huge. Emma describes how, in the midst of her daughter's illness, she would realise at 10.30 at night that she hadn't done a single thing for herself except brush her teeth since waking up in the morning. Bedtime is particularly tough. 'I'd be shattered and ask gently if she might put herself to bed, thinking to myself I just can't do any more, and even that innocuous comment would set her off.' Her daughter would start to whimper, cry piteously. 'I'd offer to watch our bedtime episode of *Modern Family* but she would be in too much of a state. Her whimper would turn to a wounded cry, then to angry screams. An hour later I am cradling her twitching form, bandaging her self-harmed wrists, singing to her like she's a baby, desperate for her to come back to me. Eventually she asks me to stop singing and I put her to bed. I am both relieved – she is no longer self-harming, she is asleep, sweet relief – but I am left feeling furious. I want to scream: "I am not happy to have to put you to bed when you are thirteen and I have spent every second of my day looking after you and I am still servicing your madness at 11.30pm. This is a shit way to live. Boring and pointless." But of course I can't say any of that. I go to sleep drained and beyond exhausted. Aware that it will all start up again tomorrow.'

As you will have gathered, parenting a teen with a mental health issue – anxiety, self-harm, an eating disorder – is an endurance test. But understanding the visceral nature and relentlessness of it, whether that's being tethered to your child during exams or comprehending the shit show it makes of a parent's life when it is more embedded, is incredibly important. If we are to support those in the thick of it, we need to understand what a grim and lonely road it can be. It is often hard to talk to friends or family about what is happening without invading the child's privacy, making it even harder to access the help we need as parents to support our sick children. Often a parents' group or family therapy can be a godsend.

But the reason I wanted to include Emma's account of what it feels like to be mothering such a teen is because as a therapist she has a great insight into what is happening inside their brains. She says that the best way to understand anorexia is that the ill brain makes a magical thinking deal with itself; when the external anxiety becomes too much, it performs a trick along the lines of: if I don't eat anything everything else will be all right. The script inside the child's head goes something like: *Now I am a teenager I feel anxious about stuff I didn't have to think about before. Like, will I manage to get some qualifications and find a job? Will I find someone I want to share my life with? What if I don't? Or, what if that boy I like doesn't like me? Am I pretty enough? Clever enough? What if I am not popular?* Their world feels out of control and terrifying; dependence on others suddenly feels very scary.

Emma says that when a teen develops an eating disorder, they have fed all these understandable developmental anxieties into the Eating Disorder Anxiety Liquidator Machine. The child makes a magical bargain in their unconscious mind which goes along the lines of: 'I can't control all of this stuff, but I can control what I eat.' But then eating anything becomes freighted with fear because the deal is that as long as you don't eat, your anxiety will go away. But of course this is not actually a sensible strategy. Not eating means that the child gets ill and depressed. The brain starts to starve. Parents notice. Doctors get involved. And the eating-disordered child is put on a meal plan, which means the parents insist that meals keep being eaten. But for the child this is a disaster because for them restricting eating is what is keeping fear at bay. It is the only control they feel that they have over anything. So telling them they have to eat is taking away their coping mechanism. Often, they say they would rather die than eat – and when they say that, they mean it. Everything is topsy-turvy. Food, the engine of life, the most basic thing a parent has to provide, becomes not homely or safe or comforting but terrifying, the enemy, because of the strange bargain they have made, that not eating will make everything okay. Ultimately, the irrationality of this thinking has to be made clear to them – but the anxiety involved in the creation of the magical thinking is centred around controlling food. They get better when they begin to see the madness of the matrix they have created for themselves, but it is a long and hard process for their parents and for them.

The good news is that most children get better. That is hard to believe for parents in the trenches, like Emma. But what I have seen from my last decade of mothering two teenage girls, and running a kind of informal sixth-form common room for all their friends, is that even those who were really bad, who became painfully thin, or were even hospitalised, are now okay. If the parents can remain solid, become like the bottom of the pool for them to push up off, then the kids seem to get better. Emma sums it up with a surprisingly English quote: 'I take comfort in British prime minister Winston Churchill's adage: "Success is not final. Failure is not fatal. It is the keeping going that matters."'

So don't be afraid of seeking help: burst into tears on your friends, get the wider family to send you regular treats. Do what you need to get through this and remember that you are loved and this too will pass.

Secret: Be the calm in the storm, the bottom of the pool for them to push up from – family therapy and professional help are your friends. Get all the support you need so you can support the ill teen. It may feel like it will never get better, but it will. I promise.

Sex, drugs – and porn

It truly is the end of an era for me. My youngest just finished her A levels and ended her school career. That means that my seventeen-year stint as a school parent – yup, all those interminable e-mails about jumble sales and assemblies and Year 10 trips and World Book Day – are now firmly in the past. That feels weird. Good. But also strange.

So what have I learnt from my decade and a half at the school gate? That it's great for kids to grow up with a stable cohort of mates in their local area. I went to school on the other side of London, it took an hour on the Tube (with my cello; I hated it and all my friends lived miles away). My kids went to school round the corner so my house is a teen hub – full of sixth-formers watching *Gossip Girl* or raiding the bagels, some even sneaking out to vape on the balcony. I know, smoking and vaping – bad, right? But I've always thought it best to pursue a strategy of radical honesty with teenagers. As a parent you either accept that they are bound to experiment and adopt a liberal approach so that they tell you what they are up to, or they lie to you. Don't think you are an exception. The parents who think their kids are angels are deluded; it's their daughters who are having sex under the swings in the local playground because they can't take a partner home. It's their sons who are hitting the chewing gum and air-freshener to hide the smell of marijuana as they head home for dinner. I've always taken the view that I'd rather the kids were under my roof, where I know, mostly, what is going on and I know who they are with; and the radical honesty policy means they can call me if they are in trouble – wherever, whenever. And, yes, that means 4am after a party or club if necessary.

I love having the teens around because that way I am immersed in their news and views; I think the future is in good hands with Gen Z. They are thoughtful, moral, kind to each other, very open in talking about what is really going on in their friendships – and they express true empathy and strength in supporting each other with their mental health issues. I know we can roll our eyes at this and murmur about snowflakes, but the mental illness epidemic among teens is real. They struggle. It's not just that it is more recognised or diagnosed either; there really is a difference in degree to how it was when we were growing up. The incidence and normality for this lot of self-harm, extreme anxiety issues and eating disorders is terrifying. In the US, the CDC's biannual Youth Risk Behavior Survey in 2023 showed that 57 per cent of teen girls say they experience persistent sadness or hopelessness (up from 36 per cent in 2011) and 30 per cent say they have seriously considered suicide (up from 19 per cent in 2011).

There is a correlation between the spike in these conditions and the advent of social media. This is the first bunch of kids to grow up constantly comparing themselves to professionally styled and digitally tweaked celebrities. Teens are always insecure. These days that natural insecurity is super-powered by the endless ping of their socials. They conduct multiple conversations with their fingers in real time; arranging, chatting, comparing – it is exhausting just watching. They are constantly camera-ready – seeing themselves through an external lens in a way that we never had to. And the FOMO (fear of missing out) is off the scale – pics from parties where they are NFI (not fucking invited) are posted in real time, and it always looks more fun than it actually is.

When it comes to sex, it has never been more important to have our communication channels open to our teens. In June 2022, in an interview with Beth Rigby for Sky News, the actress Emma Thompson encapsulated why succinctly: 'When I hear stories in schools about boys and what they expect from girls, what they think sex is, it is really disturbing,' she said. 'It can interfere with their sexual development because it's all been taken away, industrialised and fed back to them in a completely indigestible pornographic form.' It's pretty bleak out there – and very different to when we were growing up. So much so that it makes me really glad to be a Queenager, not a Gen Z.

I have been campaigning about the effects on our kids of unfettered access to internet pornography for over a decade. Then there's the impact of shows like *Love Island*, which I watch with my teens, where boys are 'players' – and the first chats they have with members of the opposite sex are about what sexual positions they like. The total pornification of sexual mores for our young people is out and proud. And it's terrifying.

Now, I am really not a prude. I was no nun as a younger woman and I frequently go into schools to talk to teenagers about sex and porn (the basic gist is that learning about sex from porn is like learning to drive by watching the *Fast & Furious* films). What is heartbreaking is how confused they all are. A marker of how much things have changed since we were young is that teen girls now think being choked is as normal a part of foreplay as a boy touching their arse or breast. Yup, you read that right. Rough, violent sex has been normalised for this generation because of the porn they watch – 90 per cent of online porn involves abuse, according to a recent French study.

I have, since 2010 when I did a cover story in the *Sunday Times* magazine called 'Generation XXX', been writing about the detrimental effect of an all-you-can-eat smorgasbord of violent sexual fantasies being available to kids with the click of a mouse without any kind of age limit or restriction. I feel a bit like Cassandra. My prophecies of kids learning about sex from porn and then enacting it, their dials set to extreme before they've even kissed anyone, have proved depressingly prescient. Many older women don't look at much of the porn that is now a pervasive influence in our culture. But I can tell you it is vanishingly rare to see a woman being given oral sex or having an orgasm. Whereas it is extremely common to see women being choked and slapped and pounded; her body just a series of orifices to be penetrated painfully, often by multiple men. To the vast majority of our young people now, this is what they think sex is. They watch porn to learn about sex and then replicate what they see there. It's why young women are almost all entirely pubic-hair-free (porn stars have no pubes). They see what we Queenagers would consider a normal pubic bush as something weird and abhorrent. The shift in sexual mores in the last decade is immense. Most midlife women never expected to have to shave off all their pubic hair (teens now think that's the norm) and when we were young, men almost never asked for anal sex. Now anal is de rigueur (third date, maybe) along with spitting in someone's mouth, being pissed on or having their pudenda spat on (this all comes from my own research in schools). I can't tell you how relieved they are when I say that sex doesn't have to be like that, that it wasn't this way for us, that sexual habits have changed hugely in a generation because of the widespread consumption and availability of hardcore internet porn.

'The biggest change in the last decade is the level of aggression girls today are encountering from boys,' explains Allison Havey, co-founder of the RAP Project, which goes into schools to talk about consent. 'It is normal now for girls to be forced, for boys to intentionally get them drunk to assault them. This generation has been bred on internet porn, which is all about violently pounding different orifices – there is no consent, no condoms, no foreplay and, terrifyingly, no sexual pleasure for women. The levels of violence are shocking and have got worse as viewers get desensitised to the material, and we're seeing all of that playing out in teen hook-ups.'

I share these stories so that Queenagers become aware of the current sexual landscape. The old rules have been thrown out of the window. But, depressingly, the double standard is still alive and kicking – you are frigid if you don't and a slut if you do. But, added to that, now there is a whole other level. If as a girl you complain about the new violent sexual mores you are seen as a Sandra Dee-style prude: it used to be a divide between girls who put out and girls who didn't. Now it is uncool to be seen as 'vanilla' when it comes to sex – cool girls are good with outré acts. And that's before we even get on to the new relationship code. This goes: if you are having sex with someone there is no assumption of exclusivity unless that is explicitly stated – so you can be sleeping with someone for six months and they can be shagging everyone else in sight and that is fine if it is an unexclusive agreement. It's what they call a 'situationship'. Of course, it's not fine. Human nature and attachment haven't changed, so the likelihood is that if you are sleeping with someone regularly you probably have feelings for them, which are not allowed in the new set-up.

The kids talk about how so-and-so 'caught feelings', as if the aim here is to have lots of anonymous, pumpy, porn-style sex rather than find someone you like and care about. If a young couple do decide to become 'exclusive' then there are lots of jokes made about the man being 'cuffed' and it is an incredibly big deal, broadcast on all their social channels. Almost like getting married.

As parents, or godparents, or aunties, we have to help our young people. The first thing we can do is talk to them about how porn is *not* sex. That sex is something you do *with* someone you like and care about, not *to* someone as part of a dare or to add a notch on the bedpost. It's important to talk to them about all of this: yes, it might be embarrassing but, no, it won't kill you. If I can go into schools and talk about this in front of 500 teenagers (on a couple of occasions, including my own teens, which made it even worse), then you can talk to just one young person whom you love.

The first thing to do is open a dialogue. Tell them what it was like for you. In my whole half-century of life, no one has *ever* tried to choke me, and I was *never* asked for anal sex. Were you? Ask them how they feel about the sexual culture around them and if they have watched porn or their friends do. Talk to the young people in your life about sex as reciprocal pleasure, about what feels good, foreplay, romance. Explain that a man should *never* hurt a woman during sex and no means no. Tell them that it is important to feel comfortable and that you trust someone before you get into bed with them. Maybe suggest they avoid copping off with a stranger after fourteen pints and two pills (sounds extreme, but it's a true story of a boy who did just that and then was accused of assault and couldn't remember what happened) for their own safety. These conversations – like the assemblies I speak at – create positive waves; they empower the girls to stop and think: hang on a minute, this didn't used to be normal ... maybe I don't have to be slapped, or strangled or have anal sex. Just telling them that it wasn't normal for us gives them tools to speak up for what they want. Kids today don't even know that what is happening to them sexually is all new and porn-influenced. They need to know that there are other ways to connect.

We can't just shut our eyes and ears to what is going on and pretend it isn't happening. Unfortunately, a hundred years of feminism haven't helped. Germaine Greer always said the sexual revolution wasn't going to be pretty. But when the advent of the contraceptive pill released women from the terror of unwanted pregnancy – meaning we could have sex just for fun, because it felt good, because we wanted to, and amen to that – I don't think any of us thought we would end up where we are now.

It's a paradox of two steps forward and one step back that Gen Z women have been told they are equal to men, educated equally, since they were born; but the boys they meet have been introduced to sex by online porn and think that is what sex is. So too many young women aren't having equal, mutually satisfying sex; they are objectifying themselves and having uncomfortable (often actively painful) sex like porn stars do. They even admit that sex for them is all about satisfying the man, and looking right, not about their own pleasure.

This has been a long campaign of mine. I've been writing and talking about the negative effects of online pornography for nearly fifteen years. It matters to me. I firmly believe that women *deserve* sexual pleasure, orgasms, to command what they want, what makes them feel good. Unfortunately, that is so not the reality. In some ways it is worse than it was when we Queenagers were growing up. When I was a teen, boys were just happy to have a real, alive girl in their bed. They didn't have a porn template. The lights went off and it was just about what felt good. Now it is all about how it looks – whether it's as 'hot' as porn. That's not progress. And nor are the increasing levels of erectile dysfunction among young men who can't get an erection with a real woman because they have become so dependent on extreme internet versions of sex.

Women deserve orgasms too! They should put that on billboards and T-shirts. Patriarchy has framed and subjugated female sexuality to suit itself, not us. The double standard is still alive and kicking – women are encouraged to have sex then discarded as sluts when they comply. Men who have many partners are studs; women who do the same are still slags. 'Madonna' and 'whore' – the archetypes at the base of relations between the sexes for the last 2,000 years – are still depressingly with us. And nothing screams 'male lens' or shows us the patriarchy in action more than porn. It's shot so the male viewer feels *he* is the one pounding the poor woman …

I've written about this countless times in all sorts of newspapers, talked about it on the BBC World Service and on TV; predicted all this would happen a decade ago. It gives me no pleasure to be proved right. But we all have to try and help fix it, and that starts with some difficult conversations.

Secret: It may feel awkward to have honest conversations about sex and drugs with the young people in your life, but if we don't talk to them about it then they will learn about sex from porn and believe that porn is sex, not a violent cartoon version of it. Tell them how it was for you. Please.

Flying the nest

It is 30 degrees, the hottest day of summer but the horse chestnuts are already autumnal brown, infected by a canker that accelerates their seasonal swap. The day feels out of sorts. I sit under a silver birch tree, sweating, as tiny yellow leaves float down in the breeze above me, dancing in the dappled sunlight like phosphorescence in a night-time sea. The grasses are golden not green, too. This seasonal mash-up is disconcerting; the hottest day of the year coupled with a fall feel. The summer finally hot after weeks of rain, as if it is having a laugh at all of us, just as the kids are back at school and my inbox is full of back-to-work woolly fashion. It's all out of whack.

But maybe that's how all transitions make us feel. Discombobulated. A bit sad. Stuck with one foot in the past and one in the future simultaneously.

Or maybe that's just how I feel. My baby is off to uni. I've been spring-cleaning her bedroom, combing with her through the accumulated stuff of her eighteen years. Her precious marble collection, the forest of furry animals who still live in her bed and an alcove. Bundles and bundles of super-neat schoolwork; commendations from her teachers, boxes of revision cards, rainbow colour-coded. So much time, so much hard work. All paying off now as we drive her to Manchester so she can start her course. There is some family hilarity that her dreams of freshers' week clubbing have been dashed by a compulsory three-day geography field trip to the Lake District – requiring a calculator, a clipboard and

waterproof trousers. She is adamant in refusing the latter, not good for
her street cred apparently. I say when the rain is lashing her freezing
legs and it's a 10-mile trudge back to her hostel she'll wish she had
them. But I won't be there, I can't insist. It's her life now.

We went on a – scorching – trip to Ikea, where, along with all the
other parents and uni fledglings, we bought saucepans and bedding,
towels and a mighty bank of plugs (so she can charge her speaker,
phone, AirPods, laptop and vape all at the same time). I veer between
feeling inordinately proud that she has made it to her uni of choice,
with her hive of mates, who have basically lived in our house for the
last two years, and feeling entirely bereft at their going. Welling up
when I think of her room empty, the house devoid of teens. It's going
to be awfully quiet around here.

And there is something bigger too. The end of a massive life phase.
We became parents nearly twenty-one years ago. Practically every day
since then we have been tending to kids' needs, making food, running
baths, picking up towels, getting them out of bed, chivvying about
homework, hanging out watching TV, going for walks. Being present,
keeping them alive. And now the everyday-ness of that is over. In its
way that is as humongous a shift as becoming a parent in the first place.

With both daughters gone, the days seem endless, luxuriant. There
is so much time for me, for us, for my work, Queenagers, my passions.
But again, that sense of having extra arms, extra caring capacity not
utilised. A bit like when I left the newspaper and I didn't know how
to slow down. It's the necessity of another change. Knowing now that
what feels strange and alien becomes normal. That slowly we adjust.
That it is difficult, but possible.

It doesn't help in the moment, though. I am easily undone by the
thought of my baby in her student kitchen, frying eggs or boiling
pasta in her new pans. Or when I clasp one of her hands – my great
delight – still endearingly squidgy even at eighteen. To hold one is
to teleport back in time; she is a toddler, standing on my lap on the

bus, her blonde curls and cheeks pressed into mine. We're playing our favourite game.

Me: 'I love you ALL!'

Her: 'I love you BIT!'

I pretend to cry and she gives me a sticky hug and shouts: 'No – silly Mummy – I love you ALL!'

We play this game over and over again. Her relishing her power. Me helplessly adoring.

I have a theory that children who have been particularly well loved have a Ready brek glow around them; a kind of undentable force field that says the world is a benign place which will greet them with a smile. That really, providing that and only that, is the true parental job. A Jamaican friend said to me: 'The love we give our children is non-conditional, it is their birthright. We love them as much as we can and we ask for nothing in return. Just the joy of giving that love, of nurturing them.' I love that. So much parental love can feel a bit conditional. We can fall into the trap of thinking that they owe us – but the truth is, they don't owe us anything. We give that love freely to propel them into the future.

I think about this as her departure draws closer – just wandering into the room full of her packed bags makes me weep. Her going is like a constant internal ache. I well up whenever I think of it. I wear my golden Queenager sunglasses like a mask to hide from her how much I mind. I don't want to burden her with my grief when she is off on her big life adventure.

I talk to friends; we whisper to each other how we feel. This secret grief for the grown-up child leaving the nest; for the end of that daily care and tending. The tears that well up, the loss of a role. My husband feels it too; I could see his eyes watering as he sat with one child either side on the sofa, hugging them tight. I know it is silly because she will come back and I am lucky to have her and no one died, and as a pal who has a differently abled child reminded me, at least mine *can* go away and live independently. Her big grief is that hers never will. Her nightmare is what will happen to her beloved autistic son when she is no longer around to love him. That he will never leave her. I know all that. I know I am lucky. But all I can say is, this sorrow is very real. Very raw.

But still. I have tools to cope. I offer up a silent prayer of gratitude for the fullness of my life. I am different from when my first daughter left two years ago. Rather than fleeing from this pain, numbing it, shutting it out, which means it erupts at the worst moments and feels overwhelming, I know now to let it flow through me. That however agonising, if I let myself really feel it, give into it, then in less than a minute it will pass. That if I move towards it, welcome the grief in with all its jaggedness, holding myself tenderly and with love, then the tears will come, but the moment will pass. I let the sadness flow through me; knowing it won't annihilate me; that grief is just love without a home. That I have felt the deepest bits of my pain before, that I know its depths, I know I can bear it. Reminding myself that this too will pass, and that grief and loss are the price we pay for love.

I attend a grief circle, run by Nicci, a friend whose mother died by suicide when she was in her early twenties. I love this woman and she me; we clicked immediately, just felt a deep familiarity. Sometimes new people turn up in your life at a particular time for a reason; we have anchored each other through huge change.

Nicci is a grief tender. She holds space for those who mourn, a most necessary task in a society that has largely forgotten the communal rituals which help us through loss. Wow, it is hard work. Sitting in a swelteringly hot room with Nicci at the front, holding the space, I hear tale after tale of losses so intense and searing I can't comprehend how these women are still standing, let alone talking. We hold a stone and speak our truths. In the circle today there is loss of parents, partners, children, friends. But also a much more nebulous and tragic kind of loss; loss of the lives the women had expected they would live.

This is extra raw around women who wanted and had not had, or could not have, children. One woman, as beautiful as a movie star, talks about being abused by her father, how it's prevented her forming the intimate partnership and family she craves. Another talks of growing up behind the Iron Curtain, with a mother who insisted she did all the housework for her four brothers (she was the only girl). She cried for the carefree girlhood she had never had, for the way that loss permeated her relationship with her own daughter; how she resented the toys, the park, the fun that her daughter has and that she never enjoyed. The bittersweetness of providing for her daughter things she had never received herself. How it throws up her own losses even as she is happy to give her child so much more.

Another talked of her dreams and ambitions being ended by ill health; the frustration of all she had wanted now being out of her reach. They wept for all that now could not be.

I had attended to support my friend and, when my turn came to share, I felt that my own grief for my baby leaving home was so trivial in comparison I almost felt embarrassed to voice it. I know that my girls need to spread their wings, that it is a sign that our job has been well done that they are flying off into their own futures. I've always loved the Kahlil Gibran poem 'On Children' about that:

Your children are not your children.
They are the sons and daughters of Life's longing for itself.
They come through you but not from you,
And though they are with you yet they belong not to you.

You may give them your love but not your thoughts,
For they have their own thoughts.
You may house their bodies but not their souls,
For their souls dwell in the house of tomorrow, which you cannot
    visit, not even in your dreams.

You may strive to be like them, but seek not to make them like you.
For life goes not backward nor tarries with yesterday.
You are the bows from which your children as living arrows are sent
    forth.
The archer sees the mark upon the path of the infinite, and He bends
    you with His might that His arrows may go swift and far.
Let your bending in the archer's hand be for gladness;
For even as He loves the arrow that flies, so He loves also the bow that
    is stable.

Sitting in the grief circle I realised that that is the task. To be the 'stable bow' – to swallow down the agony of the departure and the empty nest, to stand strong so that they can venture forth unencumbered. It is not about us and how we feel; it is about them and their journey into their hard-worked-for future. I know this, and I know that in comparison to the losses that I sat and witnessed, my loss is as nothing. But that doesn't stop it hurting any less. All endings involve loss and grief. But we have to remind ourselves that in the space that a death leaves, there is room for new things to grow, if we have the courage to see that and to let it happen. Our children are our greatest teachers. They know our weakest points and can push on them hard. But one of the great sweetnesses of motherhood is seeing them flourish and nurture in their turn, pay forward all the love that they have received.

Secret: As Gibran says – your children are not your children. They belong to the future. Our role as parents is to stand strong, shoot them forward and let them go.

PART FOUR

WORK AND PURPOSE

My midlife pivot was brought about because of work. For two and a half decades I had defined myself by my job. It was my identity, the scaffolding on which the rest of my life was built. Then suddenly it was all over. There is a terrible, falling-off-the-roof moment when you realise the life that you had, everything that you thought you were and it consisted of, is no more. It is like a death. The end of what was. There is no way back, only a scary uncertain future. We are lost in the dark, scary wood with no white pebbles to guide us out.

When that happens there is no quick fix. Sometimes this big shift is thrust upon us; other times there is a slow descent into a place where we know we aren't happy, where things get so bad that we know we have to make a change. Both are tough. This section is about navigating those times. The big disappointment or realisation and what it takes to work through them to a truly new version of you, one that neither you nor those around you might ever have expected to emerge.

And to achieve that we have to do something new, change the walls, leave behind everything we knew. Which was how, in an extremely uncharacteristic move, I found myself visiting a healer on Dartmoor. She told me many wise things and saw deeply. I am a natural sceptic – all those years weighing facts as an editor – but it was uncanny how much this woman knew about me. She kept dropping things in; that my stepfather was sending me a hug, that I had an important message to put out there, that a friendship that had come to an abrupt end really was over – that it was no longer my path. That she was tuning me up for courage – I lay among her fifty or so gongs on a raised bed as she filled me up with vibration. Can you hear the goddesses marching, she asked, as the cacophony round me swelled and intensified? It sounds bonkers, but I really could!

One story she told me was about sky burial, an ancient ritual where a corpse is left for the birds to come and pick it clean. I didn't know why she was telling me about such a seemingly barbaric custom, or how it fitted in. But she was adamant that I needed to be picked clean, to say farewell to my old life. To do that she said I would need to create an important relationship with a bird. That it was coming to me.

At the time I had no idea what she meant by that, or how it might happen. I'd never been particularly interested in our fine feathered friends. But as the months and years have unfolded since, so much of what she intimated that day has indeed come to pass. Was this the power of suggestion? Had she given me a kind of meta-narrative or perhaps permission to try thinking in a different way? I am not sure, but I do date my obsession with birds in general and especially the heron at the pond to that day. I now see that the heron has indeed helped me 'pick clean' the bones of my old life.

I didn't always like the heron much. My infatuation with him grew slowly. In the spring the pond is alive with adorable fluffy ducklings, yellow and cute. They swim after their mothers in formation, the mummy duck constantly cheep-cheeping her anxiety. There can be six or even eight ducklings in each flock. Yet the duckling population always diminishes, swiftly. One of the big culprits is my 'friend' the heron, who swoops down from above and munches them for lunch.

He is big, his wingspan four or five feet at full stretch. He stands for long periods on one leg under the trees, watching deep into the water for fish; then he lunges, popping up with silver scaliness in his mouth.

As he soars down to skim the surface of the water, he is majestic. As he scales the top of the trees, often with just one massive beat of his wings, he reveals his latent power. In myth the heron represents self-determination, self-reliance. Boundaries. He is no one's mate, he is the boss, he sits at the top of the pond hierarchy. It is his domain. Surveying us all, he balances, nonchalantly, on one leg – he stands alone.

I have become obsessed by him. I feel it is mutual. Often I will arrive at the pond and he will be absent, but as I swim out into the cold he swoops over my head, lands and seems to watch me. 'Hello, Mr Heron,' I say.

On days when he is there, I am glad. He has stalked my thoughts and my dreams. I have reams of heron pictures and cards. A friend sent me a photo of huge herons in Cape Cod, saying she saw them and thought of me. But why? Why has the heron become my totem, my spirit bird? I think it is because, as we push through these hard places, so too must we all learn some heron traits. No, *not* eating ducklings! But on this journey from what we were to what we might become, we must find inside ourselves some heron-like toughness, resilience and balance. Work out what we can tolerate and what we can't. Where we must, with self-protective ruthlessness, draw the line.

Sometimes the bones need to be picked clean, we have to make a hard, self-defensive choice to survive; sloughing off something, or someone, or a role or an identity we once cherished.

The heron for me exemplifies the kind of solitary, no-nonsense toughness that this part of the journey requires; a kind of steely determination to do the work, to see it through. No matter the pain, the sacrifice, the guilt of what our shapeshifting does to others … We will shed, and we will survive and flourish.

But first we have to dig really deep, excavate and burrow into hard places to create the change we need in order to become what we were meant to be. To shapeshift into whatever ultimate form our true nature takes.

On the scrap heap

I never expected to feel more energised, more motivated, more excited about my career and purpose at fifty-two than I ever did before. I particularly didn't expect that outcome when I sat feeling broken and rejected after being made redundant from the job I'd loved and had given my all to for nearly twenty-five years. That job had been a huge plank of my identity and, as it was so totally tied into the 24-hour news agenda, I was never really off duty. When I was suddenly terminated by a new boss, I felt like I'd been pushed off a roof, in freefall. Without the status and identity the job had bestowed upon me I felt lost, unprotected, pathetic. I felt like all my power and skills had gone with the title; like Samson when they cut his hair.

And the truth is that it is exactly at this moment, when we are most completely on our uppers, that we are expected to summon the confidence and energy to reinvent ourselves. To trot around recruiters telling them about our multiple transferable skills, all sunny and smiley, projecting the best shiny version of ourselves to get a new gig – while inside we feel wretched, humiliated, broken. I didn't even know then what my real skills were. Okay, I knew I was an editor, could string a sentence together, had run teams. But I've since learnt that my marketable skills were very different from the job spec – that, for instance, I am very good at speaking truth to power, and giving keynote speeches and chairing panels, and guiding conversations and storytelling. I've made good money as a consultant coaching

CEOs – particularly women – to sing a better song of themselves, blow their own trumpet in the most effective way, so that others can sing it when they are not in the room. I had no idea that any of those things might be useful, or that I could do them, or sell them. So often we don't know our own strengths.

Many of the women I talk to at Noon haven't chosen to opt out of work, work has opted out of them! Research from LeanIn.Org and McKinsey presented in their Women in the Workplace 2023 report found that for every woman promoted to director level, two women left. Cranfield University's survey into women on boards also finds that the number of women holding leadership executive roles has been stuck at between 12 and 14 per cent for nine years. (Yes, we now have 40 per cent of women on the top 350 UK business boards, but the vast majority are non-executive directors, they don't have the levers.) One in ten women of menopausal age (i.e. between forty-five and fifty-five) leave their jobs, according to the British Menopause Society. But our research would suggest this is not just about menopause but a combination of all the pinch points women hit at this age: divorce, bereavement, illness, tending to elderly parents, dealing with teens suffering an epidemic of mental health issues, and, of course, the elephant in the room, gendered ageism – where ageism meets sexism.

As you get to about fifty it's amazing how many women are 'let go'; often with settlements and NDAs (non-disclosure agreements), so we don't hear about it. There is a massive Queenager brain drain going on. We are leaving the workforce just as we should be storming the citadels. Being put in a walking hot-flush box, just when we should be taking our seats in the boardroom. Why else is there still such a dearth of women at the top?

Women have been entering the professions in the same numbers as men since the mid-1990s but the top echelons are still stubbornly male; across all sectors, from academia to politics, business to law firms, only approximately 15–20 per cent of top management jobs go to women. The higher you go, the more blokey it becomes – and the men circle the wagons to protect their own.

When I was made redundant just after I turned forty-nine, I realised being exited as a senior woman wasn't just personal, but systemic; that particularly in media, advertising and marketing there are vanishingly few older women left. Less than 2 per cent of the advertising/marketing workforce are women over fifty according to *Campaign* magazine. No wonder we Queenagers feel ignored/invisible in the culture (over half of us, according to our Noon survey) and little surprise that, despite people over fifty controlling 80 per cent of the wealth (Queenagers are called 'super-consumers' by *Forbes* magazine, behind approximately 90 per cent of all household consumer spending decisions in the United States, according to research by AARP), we appear in less than 12 per cent of advertising. Even though people over fifty will be the biggest consumers in *all* sectors by 2040. And our Noon research shows that university-educated women (the richest ones) would be 63 per cent more likely to buy from a brand that represents them. I know, crazy, right? When I interviewed Sheryl Sandberg (the woman who built one of the most successful advertising machines on the planet), shortly before she stepped down as COO of META, she told me that my Queenagers were 'the most lucrative and under-served cohort in the whole of the marketing firmament'.

That kind of cultural visibility matters. Hanneke Smits, CEO of BNY Mellon UK and global chair of the 30% Club, the biggest campaign for gender equity in the world (full disclosure, I am on their steering committee), has identified what she calls 'a new Queenager brain drain'. She explains that 'because of improved parental leave, women now return to their jobs after pregnancy but we are losing them at around forty-five to fifty – that matters as the average age of a female CEO is fifty-six and a female chair sixty-one. If all the senior women leave, we will never get to gender parity at the top.'

So why do Queenagers leave the jobs they love? Let's take Kate. Her story organically reflects many of the issues we found in our research. She is a highly skilled and respected producer in the creative industry. There is a redundancy package on offer, particularly for older, more expensive workers. She came to me wondering whether to take it.

She explained that she loves her job, but that after having (successful) treatment for breast cancer she's been focusing on her health and trying not to get too tired. That is tricky since on the day of the live programme she runs she regularly does a sixteen-hour day, which isn't good for her body or stress levels. Like many Queenagers, she says, 'These days, I find it really valuable just having time to walk or make supper slowly, or hang out with my two teenage children who will both be off to university in a couple of years.'

She is also responsible for her mother, who lives three hours away. Her siblings live on the other side of the world so the elder-care duties fall on her, and her mother keeps having falls and needing attention. Kate can work flexibly sometimes but says, 'I am getting a bit sick of always being on someone else's timeline and having to ask permission all the time. I'm fifty-eight, I really value my autonomy. Also, although I usually work three or four days a week – and have done for decades – I only have a two-day contract, so that is all my small pension is based on.'

This pensions gap is a massive issue for many females at this point. Women in the UK have less than half the pension savings of men by the time they reach retirement, so this scenario will be familiar to many. 'If I take the redundancy package on offer, I'll get three years' salary, which I could use to boost my pension or pay off a chunk of my remaining mortgage. I hope they would use me as a freelance and I could also get work elsewhere, so that is tempting ...'

But for Kate the biggest attraction in leaving is something I hear time and again from the Queenagers I speak to. 'Most of all I am finding it harder and harder to take instructions from people much younger and more inexperienced than me. They'll say: Let's do this. And I think, we did that twenty-five years ago, and ten years ago, and it didn't work. Yesterday I got quite cross, which is really unlike me. I don't think I can go on being polite about it and biddable; sometimes I feel my insides shrivelling, I just feel: oh no! I just can't go round that circuit again. I know that probably isn't fair and I should be more enthusiastic, maybe it will work this time … But, and it is a big but, I also think my experience should be more respected, that my track record should count for something. I'm kind of sick of being pleasing and nice when I don't agree with a decision, and I am less malleable than I used to be because on some things I know I am right and I am just not going to give way.'

That feeling of just not wanting to play a subservient role to a more senior, usually male, boss is perhaps the most common reason I hear for Queenagers wanting to quit. It's as if we get to this stage and we have the wisdom of being forged in fire, of knowing what we are talking about, and we just don't want to kowtow anymore. Women at this stage become more forthright, less worried about being 'pleasing' and liked than they were when they were younger. Essentially, if it means shutting up and putting up, we've had it with that. We just don't want to do it anymore. That sense of frustration becomes particularly powerful as a driver when it is coupled with the other massive Queenager instinct to try something new.

Part of this, as Kate expresses, is about not wanting to be so agreeable and amenable anymore. Many of us women of around fifty were raised to look after others and not complain. Which means that many women end up being what Rebecca Hill, co-author of *From Work Life to New Life*, calls 'wives to the organisation' – mentoring, doing the behind-the-scenes admin, providing the social oil, buying the staff birthday cakes, being a social 'wife' to the boss at company events, not to mention picking up all the office drudgery that keeps the wheels rolling, but never getting recognised when it is time for a promotion.

Or, as another one of my Queenagers Sarah Taylor Philips put it rather brilliantly, 'Fifty was a crazy time for me and I could never articulate which "M" it was that was responsible for tipping me over the edge. Was it my marriage, my menopause, my misery, my mental health, being a mum, my mum, my midlife crisis or money?' When we spoke, she explained to me that in fact the final straw for her was 'a mixture of *all* the Ms above, and starting not to enjoy a glass of wine because of menopause at the same time was too much. It definitely was a midlife clusterfuck.'

Sarah told me that she had lived her life a different way round from most. She'd run a successful start-up in her thirties, married and had kids in her forties, completely lost herself in her early fifties and is now in her mid-fifties and 'back in the room loud and clear and trying to get started in a corporate again. I've got so much expertise and crystallised wisdom to bring to the workplace. But currently there is no bigger narrative about what this can look like; we need to hear these stories from women who have reinvented.'

I am thrilled by that idea of being 'back in the room'. I applaud how Sarah and many others are picking themselves up again after a midlife collision. And I totally believe that we need to hear the stories of women who have reinvented, whether in career terms or elsewhere. We are a pioneering generation; we need new road maps for what this can look like.

And I love these two stories because they bring to life so much of what we found in our Noon research. How we can move into our power and find our voice in our fifties and beyond, and the necessity of that. The hunger for a new challenge, a purpose, to which we can bring everything we already know but also experience the deep excitement of learning new things, and the joy of becoming something new again, exploring unknown territory. It is that which makes us feel young again, the creation of new, salient, meaningful experiences. Doing something we haven't done before. Getting out of our comfort zone. I wrote an article about how, when I was let go at nearly fifty, I felt like I had died but now I feel like I am back in my twenties, re-energised, alive. It struck a chord with millions of readers, trending in the MailOnline for twenty-four hours over New Year's Eve 2023/4. The possibility of reinvention, of a new chapter, and the telling of those stories is massively powerful and inspirational for women at this point, because they are so rarely told.

Over the last few years I have given many talks to many corporates, and over and over again I have felt a huge disjunct between what Queenagers tell us they want from jobs and employers – to feel valued, autonomy, flexibility and control over their own time, meaningful work, purpose, to be seen – and what the corporate world tends to give older women. Ummm … status if they are still in a job (although flexibility is valued sixteen times more than status in our research) and lots of 'corporate wife-ing'.

At a landmark conference organised by 55/Redefined (who get fifty-somethings back into jobs) and the international accountancy firm EY, I got the lift down to the street with a senior female banker in her fifties. 'It felt so good this morning to feel relevant again, like someone was interested in me and what I've got to offer. To be seen … It made me realise how invisible I usually feel.'

It is not too late. We can reinvent. We've definitely got time for one more big throw of the career dice, or a shift into purpose. We can still become what we were meant to be. In fact, in our Queenager years we have the self-knowledge, experience, nous and confidence to be better employees than ever; many of us no longer have caring responsibilities so we are freer to concentrate on our work than ever. But society and employers aren't seeing it that way because of the gendered-ageist lens that is put on older women.

I never thought I'd be an entrepreneur for the first time at fifty … but now I am. What could you be? Go on, dream. What would you do if you weren't afraid? That is the first step to finding out your true passion and making it a reality.

Secret: As younger women we are pleasing, both physically and temperamentally. We put up with a lot just to be allowed in the room. As Queenagers we want purpose, to be heard, to be allowed to use our experience and power – and if we can't, we'll leave. You are not alone – dare to dream: what could you be? There is much more to come!

Extending the runway

One of the main ways in which we need to reprogramme ourselves is in how we think about our lives as a whole. We've grown up with the idea that there are three stages – childhood/education, then work and then retirement. Now, that worked just fine when we had 'but three score years and ten'. But, since science and statistics say we may well live to nearly a hundred, the old three-stage model doesn't fit anymore. I mean, do you know anyone who started doing a job or was with a company in their twenties who is still there at seventy-five? Quite.

The problem is that our society hasn't got its collective head around the 100-year lifespan yet. We're all running on the old model and then realising when we hit about fifty that we are only halfway through. That there is 'so much more to come' but we hadn't planned for it.

It's like the producer of a play coming to his cast half an hour before curtain-up and saying, 'You've got an extra forty minutes to fill, folks, the show is being extended.' Inevitably, the players panic and start padding out the third act, adding some extra speeches, elongating it. But, of course, to really get the benefit of that forty-minute dividend, it would be better to rewrite the whole script, and pace the play for the extra time.

That is exactly what we should be doing with our whole-life planning.

'It's like a dance. We've collectively learnt to dance in a three-part rhythm, think about a waltz,' explains Canadian longevity guru and super-Queenager Avivah Wittenberg-Cox. 'Now we're moving into a four-part rhythm instead, and that changes everything.'

Avivah has spent the last two decades advising corporates about gender balance, so is fluent in business-speak. She now talks about '4-Quarter Lives' (which is in fact the title of her excellent podcast); a bit like the Q1, Q2, Q3, Q4 that companies use, but she is applying the concept to a new way of thinking about different generations pulling together in the workforce and viewing the stages of our lives in a new four-part way. Avivah is passionate about the need to 'make the most of the extra decades that medical science has given us in the last century. I see this as a new road map for the long haul.'

So, what do these new quarters mean? Q1 Avivah calls 'Grow'. It stretches from zero to twenty-four. It's when we get born, parented, hit adolescence, get educated and head out into the world. It's when we learn, explore and grow in multiple dimensions, physically, relationally, intellectually.

Q2 she dubs the 'Age of Achievement'. It covers ages twenty-five to forty-nine. I suppose this is what we used to think of as typical adulthood – what younger generations now call 'adulting'. That means getting a job, living independently from our parents, settling down, finding a partner and having a family, establishing ourselves in our careers. It is all about ticking the boxes we've been given by our birth families and their expectations, jumping the fences they suggested we should. 'Q2 is often about proving oneself in the world, often in response (or reaction) to the script that's been handed down by culture, context or family,' she says.

That certainly makes sense to me. In my life, the years twenty-five to forty-nine were definitely of achievement, having two kids, getting married, buying a house, building my career in newspapers. What Avivah calls 'proving yourself to society's benchmarks' – I did that with bells on. It was overwhelmingly exhausting; I often felt like I was failing everyone as I struggled to juggle all those balls. Q2 is tough for women. 'The experience of Q2 can be very "gendered"', Avivah agrees. 'It's different for women and men, because it is women who have to carry the children and be pregnant in this time.' She is right.

I have found in the numerous talks I have given that the message that not everything has to be squished into Q2 is massively resonant for women. I wrote a newsletter called *Slow Down, Ladies, There's Time* … explaining that, in their 100-year life, women have the opportunity to power up again in terms of career or purpose later on, in their fifties or sixties, that it doesn't all have to be done between thirty and fifty. It had a rapturous response from younger women – they loved the idea of extending the runway, of not having a sell-by date. It reminded me of Oscar-winner Michelle Yeoh, age sixty, telling the world: 'Ladies, don't let anyone tell you you are past your prime.' (It is staggering to believe that she was the first female Asian actor *ever* to win an Oscar … and a Queenager to boot.)

Avivah agrees. 'My career advice for harried, stressed-out 30-year-olds is to breathe deeply, take a beat and plan for maximum impact in Q3.' Interestingly, when I spoke at a big bank about the age of achievement, several of the younger women raised their hands. 'We don't see this bit so much as being about achievement but survival,' they said. I can relate to the exhaustion of trying to cram everything into those decades, kids and career. No wonder so many millennials are voting with their feet and deciding not just that they can't 'have it all' but they don't want it! Employers should take note, younger women are not less resilient than Queenagers, they are just opting out much earlier on! There is a whole new 'Lazy Girl', work-to-live attitude out there. Younger generations don't see why they should just keep grinding away, and in turn are more confident about finding other, alternative routes of income. If organisations want to hang on to this generation, they need to start role-modelling how good it is to be a senior woman in their company, so that there are women for these younger cohorts to look up to. I have spoken to many HR directors who are worried about their leaky female pipeline. Queenagers are the canaries in the coalmine for getting it right for the women coming up behind.

Extending the runway of women's careers into their Queenager years – our prime – doesn't just help midlifers, but would particularly help women at this point not feel like they have to stuff everything in. Maybe they will then actually be able to remember those years. My own 'survival' years, when I had tiny kids and an enormous job, are just a blur of exhaustion. It should have been the time of my life – professional and family success. But the reality was just knackering. I lost myself.

It is the next life segment – ages fifty to seventy-four – what Avivah calls Q3 and I think of as our Queenager years, that is the new and crucially important piece of this 4-Quarter/100-year life jigsaw. Avivah and I both think of this phase as the time of 'Becoming'. I say on Noon that fifty is when we become the women we always wanted to be. She concurs, saying that Q3 is an entirely new phase, where we really see the benefits of longevity and the fact that, if we can stay healthy, active and engaged, we can have a fulfilling time well into our seventies and beyond.

She cites studies by management guru Peter Drucker, which show that almost 40 per cent of the US labour force is currently over fifty (by 2030, 47 per cent of the UK labour force will be fifty-plus too). But most companies have not woken up to this fact. 'Where we are now on age reminds me of when I first started my work on the importance of gender balance twenty-five years ago.' The two are of course linked. After all, we're never going to get to gender parity at the top if all the women leave at fifty. Tackling gendered ageism and keeping Queenagers on track with their careers are crucial if we are going to shift the dial.

'This rethinking of our longer lifespan and what that means in terms of work, relationships and society is just beginning,' Avivah explains, adding that a good Q3 needs careful planning and thought.

'If we are to dance into it gracefully then we need to have done the groundwork. That means changing the way that we think about our lives and recognising that Q3 is a thing, that it is coming our way and to prepare for it early.'

It is clear that for many the shift from Q2 into Q3 can be bumpy. For me the big pivot at fifty, the beginning of Q3, was professional, out of a corporate and into purpose and entrepreneurship. In doing that, I also realised that much of my Q2 drive had come from fulfilling the 'achievement at all costs' wishes that had been programmed into me by my birth family.

For Avivah, the big into-Q3 pivot was more personal. She left her husband, her home and the life she had built in France, and broke up her family to move to London and marry a new husband. 'It was the hardest thing I have ever done. It involved huge amounts of pain and fallout – but that shift is what made me, me. It is having the courage to make those big changes that helps you create your Q3. It is the essence of becoming. I think of this Q3 phase as being intrinsically driven, i.e. coming from inside us, rather than externally driven.'

At fifty we finally slough off everyone else's expectations, all that family and cultural conditioning, and go: this is me. If you don't like it, sod it, because I do like it. It feels like my new shape. It feels like the woman I always wanted to be. It is in Q3 when we become Queenagers that we come into our prime. Q3 is when you shed stuff; it is the joy of ageing, when you truly don't give a stuff and reach for the stars.

Of course there is a caveat. Q3 builds upon Q2. I had options as a Queenager because of the experience, money and family I had built up during those years of achievement/survival. I am afraid there are structural inequalities here which reflect the unfairness of life. 'If in Q2 you have no money and no pension and no partner, then Q3 will be harder. There are deep divisions here depending on our achievements in Q2 and, of course, where we started in Q1.' A massive study by the Institute for Fiscal Studies found that intergenerational inequality is increasing; that for Gen Y their level of wealth and attainment and whether or not they are home owners is much more closely linked to parental wealth than it was for those born in the 1960s. Of course, the financial resources we have, combined with our education and personal circumstances, all play a huge part in what is possible in terms of Queenager Q3 reinvention.

Having her family spread all over the world is not easy for Avivah. 'How we gather everyone and weave links together is tricky but I do see that as my role as a modern matriarch.' That idea of 'gathering' the family being a Queenager duty and indeed the very notion of a modern matriarch is music to my ears. Avivah's problem is where to do that; she feels a strange sense that her family now has no central point. 'With my mother passing it is like a second empty nest moment – that feeling of having to do something, look after someone, and realising that actually you don't because they are no longer there. To get through the loss you just have to breathe and slow down and be kind to yourself. Trust that the next phase will emerge.'

Avivah's Q3 present to herself – and it is a trend we see often in the Noon community – was to go back to study, in her case at the prestigious Elders Academy at Harvard University. 'I loved being a student again, it was so liberating and so much fun! I feel strongly that when you are through with working you are through. Period.' While there she worked on her 4-Quarter Lives thesis, which is now the basis of her work and bestselling *Elderberries* Substack. 'We all have to go on learning new things, stay flexible and engaged. It was a heady bit of reinvention; I met so many inspirational people in their sixties and seventies who were all busy starting new chapters too. We all want to push our Q3 for as long as possible.' Amen to that!

Eventually, though, Q3, the time of becoming, comes to a close – although for many of us, if we have a good healthspan, it can continue into our eighties. But at some point we all hit Q4 – which Avivah has dubbed 'Harvesting'. Though when I told my dad about that he guffawed and said, 'It's not harvesting, it's dying!' Which made me laugh, although maybe it shouldn't have!

But in some ways my dad is right. In our Western cultures we've lost our models of aspirational death. In the West we've tried to eliminate death entirely from our lives, losing the rituals and traditions about how to do it well and how to support others in grief. 'But, of course, before we get to our dying it's about living, and in Q4 we reap the benefits of all we have spent a lifetime sowing and the most important thing is to keep on growing. For those who have sown well this is a time for legacy, giving back, grandparenting and purpose. For too many it can bring loneliness and poverty and despair. So all the more reason to plan wisely now.'

I love Avivah's ideas on how we can rethink our lives, reprogramme our expectations for the long haul, for the longer lifespan that we are lucky to live. Naturally, transitions are tough; I began this book by talking about how change is difficult. But if we understand the challenges and shifts to come, we can make them easier for ourselves. For instance, I was with a friend who, in her early fifties, three or four years before her children left for university, retrained as a counsellor. She now runs creative writing groups where the participants use poems to talk about transition, or grief. Her work is fulfilling. 'My kids are leaving home and I thank God that I started this new work, this new purpose for me before they went, so I have something I am passionate about to fill my days.' As the old Royal Marines maxim goes: Prior Preparation and Planning Prevents Piss-Poor Performance. PPPPPPP ... it is true in life as well as war.

Secret: In the 100-year life, fifty is only halfway through. If we are going to make the most of our increased lifespan then we have to be strategic about what the next quarter will require and start planning early.

The Queenager brain drain

We've heard about the Queenager brain drain. It's real. Women aged forty-five and over are leaving the workplace in unprecedented numbers. A new report by EY calls the phenomenon 'the disappearing women'. Over the last few years I have been talking to companies about how to retain their Queenagers; after all, we will never get to parity at the top if senior women leave just as they are poised to conquer the higher realms of management. In my old company, becoming a senior executive used to be referred to as 'entering the death zone', because once you are in the C-suite or just below, career termination can come at any point … The air is thin, all it takes is a change of boss and everyone in the marzipan layer (just below the icing) becomes vulnerable. But the sheer rate of exodus of Queenagers at this point is more than natural wastage. And stopping the exodus of senior women really matters.

The FTSE 100 in the UK has around eight female CEOs; in the US it is similarly around 10 per cent in the US Fortune 500. According to the most recent research by Cranfield/Women on Boards, in the big executive jobs the figure is stuck at around 14 per cent, although there are now more non-executive directors who are women, that number increasing from 12 per cent to 40 per cent in the last decade. But to some extent that is window-dressing when the roles with the real power, the ones controlling the levers, remain stubbornly male.

So what is going on? Why, after battling valiantly up the slippery corporate pole for twenty-five or even thirty years, are we seeing so many Queenagers throwing in the towel? And remember that this cohort have resilience running through them like a stick of rock – we began in what a top lawyer friend of mine called the 'hand on the ass' days. We Queenagers are used to toughing it out.

Well, the higher you go, the blokier it gets. I've heard chilling stories of women on boards who discover that there is a secret male WhatsApp group where the real business gets decided. Or that all the decisions have already been agreed during a round of golf or some after-dinner drinks (sometimes at an all-male club, or strip bar) where the woman wasn't invited. This is not ancient history; it is still happening now. In the UK, the top business organisation the CBI, or Confederation of British Industry, was rocked by a series of sexual harassment scandals, a culture of *droit du seigneur* where groping of younger females was common. It's not just the old dinosaurs, either; the bro culture of Silicon Valley also operates in a way that excludes women from the tech frontier companies which are the architects of the AI future we will all inhabit. The dearth of women at the top of business and broader leadership matters to us all.

While the lower orders of businesses are more egalitarian, at the top it is very much still a man's world. Many of the women who make it there do so by becoming men in skirts; one woman I knew who became a CEO talked solidly about cricket and football and did military fitness workouts at the weekend. She also shut down every female-friendly initiative that was ever established (on the grounds that it was 'sexist' to men, a surefire way of keeping in with the senior men but not great for the other women in the organisation). These leaders look like women, sure – but are they bringing anything different to the role if they become just like, or even worse than, the blokes when they get there? Often these women have got there by defining themselves as exceptions, different or better than other women. It's classic queen bee syndrome. I once congratulated a powerful businessman on appointing a female

CEO. When I subsequently bumped into her at a party I discovered she was furious. 'Don't *ever* remind my boss that I am a woman,' she said. 'It's much better if he forgets that fact.' Ouch. So much for women leading differently!

As well as the difficulties of surviving the boys' club, the flexibility that our research revealed is important to Queenagers (more so than status) is often hard to come by at the top of a company. Leaders tend to have to be in the office five days a week and on call 24/7 in those kinds of extreme jobs, which is tricky for Queenagers being hit by the midlife clusterfuck. And there is something else here too. After twenty-five or thirty years in the corporate world, women have options, they can vote with their feet. Our research found an overwhelming sense of Queenagers feeling they'd had enough of being a square peg in a round hole, of playing the game. Or, as Kate put it in an earlier chapter, being 'pleasing'. Meaning and purpose also become more important to us at this stage. As well as that sense of, I'm fifty, I might not have that much time left, I want to make it count. And many are just tired of managing up. Or managing the egos and macho psychopaths who famously proliferate at the top of organisations.

Take Thelma's story. I went to meet her for a coffee after she had agreed her exit from the company she worked for. She was the second most important person in the company and, in the short time she was there, nearly thirty women left because of the intense misogynistic bullying of the CEO.

As soon as Thelma got her feet under the desk, she discovered the problem was far worse than she had been told. 'I realised there were zombie departments where there would be four people being paid but only one was ever in the office and three were off on long-term "sick leave" – i.e. had been subjected to such bad bullying by the boss that their mental health was so affected they could no longer work.' When she tried to talk to HR she found they were so scared of the CEO that they did not want to be seen to be talking to her, and it got to the point where if she wanted to talk to the head of the department she had to do it in secret either off site or on Zoom on her rare days at home.

Thelma is no shrinking violet; she has worked in the construction industry for twenty-five years but this boss, she said, was 'so sadistic that he was seen to skip across the office with a huge grin on his face when he had publicly torn yet another person to shreds'. He didn't just do this to women; Thelma described how one of his senior male reports shook after a brutal dressing-down. 'The boss thought he was engineering "creative chaos"; actually, he was just destroying the efficacy of the organisation. And yet because he had been hand-picked by the proprietor, he was untouchable – despite all the "inclusive" guff on the organisation's mission statement about how they were a wonderful, equitable, inclusive employer. I've seen that so often in my career, the "rock star" men who are seen to bring in the clients, or the revenue, are allowed to get away with murder, despite endless inclusion and behaviour policies.'

It was women, however, who really riled him. He would regularly tell Thelma that the women in her department were not just useless but insane and incompetent. He would banish women from meetings and ostracise them by berating any other member of staff he saw talking to them.

'In some of the meetings he chaired he would pick on the most junior woman in the room and just interrogate them about something trivial until they cried or were shaking with fear and shame.' Thelma started off by trying to defend her staff but the CEO would become so irate it was impossible. The senior women he hired he saw as 'a bit like girlfriends; to begin with they would be flavour of the month, but then he would start undermining their authority, negating decisions they had made, or they would be excluded from key meetings, or told a project that they thought had the go-ahead was now not happening. It was a culture of gaslighting and fear.'

Thelma noticed how all the men around him would start to subtly ape his mannerisms or dress; he wore a particular shade of cream shirt and she realised that all the other men in his meetings were wearing exactly the same hue. He was a classic case of only trusting 'mini-mes', only seeing competence in other jockish, Ivy League men from wealthy backgrounds, frat-boy types who wore a sheen of total confidence at all times, 'usually erroneously' in Thelma's view. 'It was amazing how often these men, who were often not qualified, were promoted over competent, experienced women. He particularly had it in for any woman who had to leave to collect a child from school or relieve a childminder; he couldn't stand them having something else in their life which was more important than him or his whims.'

As we have seen recently with many corporate male leaders, he was obsessed about his employees being in the office, not 'ditching', as he put it. 'The company needed to change but, because he was such a control freak and insisted that everything went through him, it was impossible to flatten the hierarchy enough to empower more junior people to make their own decisions. When I tried to point this out to him, he became so angry – bright red and huffy – I had to leave the room. When I complained to HR about the number of women who had left, they just shook their heads and said there was nothing they could do.'

Thelma was clearly distressed by the experience when we met. Her hands shook, and her skin was grey. She blamed herself for taking the job and giving the boss the cover of having made a senior female hire in the first place. 'I should have realised there was a problem as soon as I arrived. In my first few weeks, some senior women who had been holding the fort came into my office and resigned; they said they couldn't be human shields anymore.' All her female colleagues told the same tale of being constantly undermined and living in a state of terror – they'd talk about their hearts racing when they got an e-mail from the boss, and waking up in the morning with dread about going into work, having lost all their confidence. In our Noon Circles I have heard versions of this exact story so often; it is shocking how prevalent this kind of sexist bullying is.

Thelma tried to shield her team, but as her relationship with the boss deteriorated she realised 'that I was only there to give a veneer that there were senior women at the top (my job had been called "the ejector seat")'. In the end Thelma realised her presence was just helping to prop up his toxic regime. She was put on gardening leave on full pay.

This is such a familiar tale to me. I've lost count of the number of formerly senior executive women who have been through a similar scenario and then even been silenced with NDAs if they want to keep their settlement. Thelma described herself as 'heartbroken at having to leave a job and an industry I love'. Additionally, she knows how hard it will be to get a similar high-profile role in her fifties.

Although Thelma's story is particularly extreme, I am sad to say it is not uncommon. At least Thelma wasn't sexually assaulted or fired on a technicality without any compensation. In our Noon focus groups we hear so many tales of women 'leaving' like this, being 'volun-told' they were taking redundancy, or walking because the pressure of juggling the midlife maelstrom and the unforgiving corporate world became unbearable. Many like Thelma express huge grief at turning their backs on careers which have defined them and are bitter about 'so-called diversity, equity and inclusion policies which sit in drawers and which don't mention anything about age or gendered ageism anyway'. Many Queenagers echoing Thelma just said they had done too many years of being 'handmaidens' or 'deputies' to more senior men; making them look good, being their 'office wife', fixing their problems. Even more were sick of the politics and the brown-nosing and having younger, less experienced, less competent often boss-mini-me men promoted ahead of them.

'I know what I am doing, I have won prizes in my industry, why should I prop up someone less good and talented than me?' said one Queenager. 'I'm off to set up my own company.' She now very profitably sells her consultancy services back to her old industry. 'I don't have to deal with any wankers, I work when I want to. I set my own prices and I take the summer off ... and, best of all, I don't have to run all my best ideas by a phalanx of senior chaps who don't get it.'

Another Queenager who has also just left a big job in financial services described how she had been working in investment banking, one of the sectors of the economy with a particularly vicious gender pay gap and few females in senior jobs, since 1992. She'd had three kids and got an MBA when they were small while also working a full-time job. (That sort of resilience is typical of the kind of women I've been talking to.) Her qualifications enabled her to get promoted and she wound up as the most senior woman in the bank, working in a team of twelve as the only female. 'I'd long learnt to tolerate the back-slapping culture – Christ, it's the price of entry in this world. If you got all miss-ish, you don't even get in the room. It's water off a duck's back to me after so long. But I worry about the younger women, they are not so resilient, which in some ways is a good thing; they just won't tolerate that kind of macho culture, but I'm not sure what will happen to them because the culture in these kinds of cut-throat banks isn't changing.' She explained that she had always tried to be 'one of the lads', but after thirty years the unfair bonus culture, extortionately high targets and incredibly long hours and back-biting simply became too much. 'I just don't need to do it anymore. It's not my first rodeo. I've earnt enough money to be able to set up my own outfit and call my own shots. I just thought, I'm fifty-four – what is life for? Enough is enough!'

This woman said that although the CEO was very encouraging of her and the other women who had made it up through the ranks, the supportive coaching they were offered had to be done during office hours and, since her work was client focused, she would do the coaching in her breaks and after work, which ended up being even more exhausting. 'In the end 40 per cent of the women in the company left. The CEO was supportive – but below the C-suite, in middle and senior management, it was still an old boys' network culture, with lots of sexist behaviours needing to be addressed. We'd just had enough.'

I hear this refrain often. Senior women saying that the corporate world is still set up for and run by, and in the image of, men; that despite women entering the workforce and the professions in the same numbers as men in the 1980s and 1990s, we are still only seeing 15 per cent of women, or less, making it to the top.

Many Queenagers come to the realisation that the only way to get the kind of freedom they crave is to run their own business. But that is also a tricky ask – 90 per cent of new businesses fail. And while going it alone works for some Queenagers (older entrepreneurs are twice as likely to be successful) and it means that individually these women get a better quality of life, it doesn't fix the systemic problem. We'll never get to parity at the top if all the senior women leave. And without equality at the top, we'll never get more representative companies and cultures. Christine Lagarde, President of the European Central Bank, who was MD of the International Monetary Fund in the wake of the 2008 financial crisis, blamed male groupthink at the top of global financial institutions for the failure of the Lehman Brothers bank. 'As I have said many times, if it had been Lehman Sisters rather than Lehman Brothers, the world might well look a lot different today.' As Lagarde, a phenomenal Queenager herself, recognised, when it comes to mitigating risk, Queenagers are the answer: experienced, tough women who speak truth to power. But gendered ageism, the midlife collision and what has been termed 'The Revolt' (Queenagers wanting to move into purpose and run their own ship and not deal with the bullshit anymore) are driving them out just when they should be taking up the reins of power.

This really matters because when Queenagers leave organisations, the tip of the arrow of social change goes with them. After all, when these women, who have been lobbying for flexible work, flatter management and generally more humane organisations since they entered the workforce at the end of the 1980s, give up, some of that drive for change goes with them. This matters because Queenagers are the canary in the coalmine when it comes to culture in organisations; a company that hangs onto its senior women is also the company with a culture that will attract the best millennial and Gen Z talent. Our Noon research into what professional women aged forty-five to sixty seek from their employers (conducted with Accenture in 2022) shows that Queenagers want decent line management; a positive culture; to be appreciated; autonomy, flexibility, respect, purpose – exactly what younger generations are after too. The problem is that when Queenagers leave they deprive organisations of important social resources – senior women are 68 per cent more likely to mentor and support junior diverse talent according to LeanIn.Org/McKinsey research. They are often the cultural glue, the institutional memory, the ones who bring in the birthday cakes and the leaving cards, the ones who make it feel like somebody cares. When Queenagers get whacked, that goes too. 'The trouble is,' says Tamara Box, managing partner of Reed Smith, a global law firm, 'the younger women are less tolerant than we Queenagers; they won't put up with it. They are quitting even earlier, which means we don't have a pipeline of younger female talent coming through the ranks. We need companies to value Queenagers and nurture the next generation of female leaders, but despite the rhetoric too often that just isn't happening.'

We Queenagers are a pioneering generation; the first cohort to enter the workforce in equal numbers to men in the late eighties and early nineties. Many of us have stuck it out, doing thirty-plus years in our professions and have got pretty near to the top; but we're getting spat out, or leaving, because fundamentally business and big organisations are still structured by and for men. The most important factor in whether a woman leaves or stays, according to law firm Clifford Chance's study with Encompass Equality, is the level of support offered by her line manager. If the line manager is unsupportive a woman has a 64 per cent chance of leaving, compared to 38 per cent on average. A toxic culture means a woman is twice as likely to leave in the next two years and this increases with age – only 38 per cent of women feel optimistic about their progression prospects in their forties compared to 65 per cent of women in their twenties. And that's before true gendered ageism really kicks in at around fifty. I saw it in the figures of a huge UK company: between the ages of 40–45 and 45–50, women made up 28 per cent of the workforce. But between 51–55 the number plunged to 20 per cent. This is the Queenager brain drain. Most companies aren't even measuring this crucial intersection of gender and age.

What's shocking is the fact that older women quitting or being whacked is simply not being talked about. I hear that over and over again. They left, or were made redundant, and nobody cared; it wasn't discussed, there was a deafening silence. The water just closed over them. Lots of businesses talk about diversity and inclusion and the need for gender parity, but there is a kind of myopia about the decimation of older female talent in organisations – it is not even measured. Don't believe me? Just ask the company you work for if they know how many women over fifty they have in the organisation and how many have left in the last two years.

Out there is an expectation that older women will just disappear, silently and without making a fuss. Well, I say enough! Queenagers matter. We've hung in there and put up with enormous amounts of shit just to be in the room. As younger women we were harassed and brutalised and simply expected to suck it up and get on with it if we wanted to stay in our jobs. As mothers – if we had kids – we were expected to work the double shift and pretend we were equal to the men, even though we were doing our jobs with the handicap of a whole other domestic job as well. Now in our fifties we are either dismissed as menopausal and 'hot' and emotional and past it; or seen as the past not the future; or not seen at all – just dismissed by the patriarchal culture as no longer even being worth consideration because we are no longer 'pleasing' in both senses. So we leave, or we set up our own outfits. And so far we haven't made a fuss.

Lucy Ryan, my colleague and author of *Revolting Women: Why Midlife Women Are Walking Out*, talks about how 'the closer the woman gets to power, the more urgent the need to put them down' – interesting in terms of all these women leaving just as they get to the top of their organisations. The brilliant Sylvia Ann Hewlett, economist and gender campaigner, talks about the men 'circling the wagons' at the top. It's still happening and the current corporate focus on menopause, although welcome in terms of health equity and protection for the 25 per cent of women who have a terrible time, also puts Queenagers back into a hot-flush biological box just as they should be being taken seriously as future leaders. No wonder it has been adopted with alacrity by so many companies! When we surveyed our Noon community, we found that over three-quarters of the women did not want to be viewed through a menopausal lens and agreed with the statement: We are Queenagers, not walking hot flushes!

Of course, it's good that menopause is no longer a taboo subject and doctors are now being given mandatory training in the symptoms (that didn't happen until 2021 in the UK, and hats off to Carolyn Harris MP and campaigners such as Kate Muir and Davina McCall, who have driven this conversation), but seeing midlife women only through that menopausal biological lens is not helpful. My worry with the increased focus on menopause is that Queenagers will get put in a hysterical, hormonal box just when in reality they are freed from monthly menses and caring responsibilities. This part of Q3, the fifty to seventy-four years for working women, should be when they come into their prime – new research from neurobiologist Dr Louann Brizendine in her book *The Upgrade: How the Female Brain Gets Stronger and Better in Midlife and Beyond* shows this. But that is still not the cultural view of older women. This is why I am so passionate about challenging the gendered ageism that saturates our culture. We need a serious Queenager programme to keep women on track in work. Only then can we reach parity in leadership and change the world. Something needs to change and quickly; on current trends it will be 136 years before women and men share the top jobs equally. Who wants to wait that long?!

It's time to stop the quiet drawing down of blinds on Queenager careers. We need to shout about this silent tragedy. Queenagers have suffered to get to where they are; it's not morally right or good for business to have a second brain drain of female talent when women hit forty-five. It doesn't make sense! It is also a problem in terms of the growing gender pension gap. Women have 35 per cent of the pension pot that men do and yet we live longer. If we are to avoid penury in old age, governments *need* Queenagers to work. Queenagers are 'super-consumers'; Lisa Edgar, Chief Insight Officer at Saga, calls them 'chief consumption officers'. They are a crucial consumer group. Companies need employees who understand them and can sell to them. Yet less than 10 per cent of advertising targets this demographic and over half of Queenagers feel invisible to brands and unrepresented in the wider culture. More broadly, older women are the fastest-growing cohort in the workforce (7 million in the UK alone) – and the global economy is facing a looming skills shortage. The world needs us to use our talent and experience and stay in our jobs; so why are so many of us being allowed to leave/forced out? When I founded Noon I had two ambitions when it came to Queenagers and work. The first was to get the corporate world to value and hang onto their senior women; the second was to get organisations to recognise the power of the Queenager consumer.

Secret: Shout it from the rooftops, please! Women over fifty make up a quarter of the population. We are super-consumers and a key talent pool. We matter. Yet we are being failed both as consumers and employees. We need a Queenager revolution.

Breadwinning and the pension gap

One of the most toxic aspects of Queenager programming manifests in the way too many of us think about money. Our Noon research reveals a worrying combination of fear and boredom as the top emotion when it comes to our finances. I know only too well the paralysis mixed with terror that accompanies chaining oneself to the desk to tackle the annual tax return. Or the way my usually fertile brain goes cloudy when I have to think about life insurance or pensions, or the mortgage.

Yet this reluctance to engage has real-life consequences. The gender pension gap for Queenagers is startling: the average British woman aged sixty-seven has £69k in pension while the average man has £205k at the same age. That is a terrifying differential, particularly since women live longer. And a third of women have no personal pension at all and a quarter of women stopped paying into their own pension while on parental leave. These trends are replicated globally.

Baroness Helena Morrissey, Noon Advisory Board member, founder of the 30% Club and ex-CEO of an investment bank, attributed this lack of retirement funds or financial planning for many women to a female reluctance to put their own future needs first. 'What is clear is that women need to push for the financial impact of family choices to be shared equally at home; women need to have frank conversations with partners about how they share the financial impact of caring responsibilities and taking time out from careers. And it is not just about caring; single women also take a big financial hit – it is more expensive running a solo household than living with someone else.'

We women need to take our heads out of the sand, stop being polite and get a grip on our money and what we need to do with it in order to have a financially comfortable old age. Particularly since we live nearly a decade longer than men so we have more time to fund. Too many of us grew up thinking that a man was a financial plan; that if we played our cards right someone else would take care of us – a legacy from our mothers' generation. Well, I'm sorry, ladies, but it's the twenty-first century, we aren't princesses in a tower and the cavalry aren't coming. If we don't do it for ourselves then nobody will.

Just look at the demographics. Around 40 per cent of Queenagers are living alone. Of those who are with a partner, over half are the main breadwinner in their households. I have always been the main earner in my marriage. It's why I've had the career I had. I've seen so many bright peers have their professional lives derailed by having a more successful husband whose job came first. Whereas in my case, because it was my salary that paid our mortgage, if the kids were sick my husband stayed at home. It was a pressure being the main breadwinner, the great provider, but also a boon. Just look at the statistics: 55 per cent of women didn't return to full-time work after the birth of their first child (compared with over 95 per cent of men). Moreover, almost half of women have had their career and finances impacted by caring responsibilities other than parenting (e.g. elder care, or caring for grandchildren) – 15 per cent gave up work, 18 per cent cut their hours, 14 per cent said there was a financial hit to them for providing care. This is a particular issue for older women. We also know there is an epidemic of divorce hitting women in their fifties. This can be a financial disaster; on average women have 35 per cent of the pension pots that men do – but for divorced women their spouse's pension pot is worth, on average, £205,800, while the woman's is a meagre £26,100 … a staggering difference of £179,700. So, if you are getting divorced,

please go for the pension not the house! In fact, if you take just one bit
of advice away from this book, make it that one.

In the many workshops for Queenagers I run, there always comes
a moment where there is a collective gasp when they realise they should
have prioritised their own future financial welfare earlier. That living
the 100-year life is all very well, but it also needs paying for. The first
step is for us, as a group, to get our heads out of the sand – say goodbye
to the ostrich – and get to grips with our own financial position. I've
run numerous Queenager finance workshops on what I call 'Queenager
financial Spanx' (the underpinnings that support our lives). The first
thing I ask the women to do is a recce. Write a list of everywhere you
have worked where you might have a pension pot. Then gather them all
together in one place. If you have defined benefits on any of the plans,
hang onto them carefully. Otherwise, it's a good idea to consolidate
your various pots to avoid extra fees. Second, do you have a mortgage?
How much longer are you paying it for? Do you have a rainy-day fund
for if you lost your job? (Or, even better, what my friend Hannah calls
a 'Fuck It Fund' – a stash of cash that means you can walk away from
a job if someone is treating you badly. She is a freelance and says this
is an essential!) Do you have a will? Life insurance? A lasting power
of attorney for if you become mentally unfit? I know all of this sounds
terrifying, none of us want to think about becoming infirm, but if
we don't want to have a penniless old age, it is also necessary. Helena
Morrissey recommends an approach to financial fitness similar to the
one we are encouraged to take for physical fitness: the mantra is 'little
and often'. Exerting agency over all of this is surprisingly satisfying;
know your position and then you can make it better. It also helps with
the anxiety factor.

I believe passionately that we need to start talking to our daughters
about this early on. All young women should set up a pension pot in
their twenties and start paying into it, even if it is only a tiny amount
a month. Then compound interest can work its magic. We need to

start telling better stories to women about the advantages of thinking early about the future. Currently the financial industry blinds us with jargon and incomprehensible spreadsheets (to me anyway). We need to tell stories about what particular financial decisions have meant for particular women and pass on good advice such as: if you get a bonus, put some of it in your pension, it's tax-free. Or if you get a pay rise, also ask for an increase in the amount your employer pays into your pension. Men ask for that kind of thing all the time – women, not so much! It's why that gender pension gap is so stark. Or if you have some spare cash, put it in an account that pays interest. That sounds so basic but I for one am guilty of not doing it; it took my daughter's boyfriend to point out what an idiot I was being and make me shift to an account with a better rate. The bottom line is that we need to put on our Queenager big-girl pants and get to grips with all of this. It's all very well having great plans for our prime, our third quarter, our new chapter – but we need the financial Spanx, the solid underpinnings, to make that vision a reality.

One of the only bits of sensible financial planning I have ever done is to pay into Child Trust Funds for my daughters. They were introduced by Tony Blair's government – every kid born on or after 1 September 2002 was eligible for a £250 voucher from the state to be invested so they had some funds when they hit eighteen. It was made very easy to augment the state funds. I took out a direct debit from my salary when my daughters were born and religiously paid £50 or £100 a month into their accounts. I am so glad that I did. This summer my eldest has been off working in a surf hostel in Portugal (some of it financed by her Child Trust Fund) and if she wants to do a master's or go travelling after she finishes uni, she'll have those options because of the saving that I did over all those years. Same with the little one – I see it as their 'follow my dreams' fund. That feels a much more persuasive reason to take up a saving habit than dreary columns of compound interest. I bet far more women would save if there was a better story told about what it would allow them to do, particularly if we tied it to new stories about what women are capable of after fifty. Currently only 15 per cent of independent financial advisers are female – and I hear over and over again how women have not been communicated with about their financial decisions in a way that makes sense to them. One of the questions I am asked most often is whether I have a good financial adviser and whether I can recommend them; and this from friends who work in financial services. Even if they are professionally financially literate, women can be ostrich-like about their own money. That has to change.

Another reason to get a grip on our money is because it matters. We Queenagers control huge amounts of wealth. We have earnt our own money but we are also inheriting it, with trillions bequeathed to Queenagers by the Baby Boomers and Greatest Generation. If we understand the power we have, we can use it to make the world a better place. For instance, when I consolidated my pensions into one, I switched it out of fossil fuels into renewables and impact funds that support female entrepreneurs. We can use our collective Queenager capital to do good. Particularly to become part of the sisterhood economy where women intentionally try to spend their money on other female-founded businesses, or invest in other women founders. We can use the power of the Queenager Pound to change the world – if we want to. If we think about it and can be bothered.

The truth is that, when it comes to our money, we can have agency if we choose to take it. It's just that, as with so much of the other programming we have inherited, it is not what we were told to do. Our generation was raised to please, to think of others, to abnegate ourselves for the needs of others. Just think of how we were conditioned in Brownies never to seek praise for ourselves, but to get on with serving others quietly, without requiring recognition. No wonder we haven't put our own financial security first … we were actively told to put everyone else's needs before our own. And as with so much of this Queenager tale, this massive shift towards women having to take control of their own finances is startlingly new. It's not our fault. We really are pioneers. When my parents got divorced in the seventies, even though my mother was a university lecturer she wasn't allowed a mortgage in her own name, she needed a male guarantor. That is still true in other parts of the world such as Saudi Arabia. It's pretty recent, only a generation, that women have taken the reins on their own finances. Many of us female breadwinners are the first women ever to take on that role. Like all things Queenager, we are breaking new ground – so it's not surprising that it is a bit of a hurdle for us to jump. But we can do this. Slow and methodical, taking agency, not being deflected, are the key. This really matters as so many women have not put their own financial futures first and, since women live longer, are facing penury in old age. We have to tell better stories to women now and the next generation so they don't face the same fate.

Secret: I know it is boring and scary but get a grip on your finances. If you have a pension or pensions, consolidate them. Work out how much money you are going to have to live on in the future and, if necessary, start saving some more. When it comes to cash, knowledge is power.

Shift into your power

I am constantly astonished by the amazing women who reach out to me on LinkedIn. One of the best of them was Lalita. I loved her posts, such as: 'You will know when you have found your purpose because it compels and enables you to swim effortlessly *with* the tide.' Or how she wrote about being a woman of colour in the tech industry with such grace, and how embracing the new, particularly anything digital, has been her secret to unlocking success. She told me how, as a young producer and reporter of colour in TV, she was usually given the worst, most boring stories. The ones with no guest to invite into the studio, no visuals. She'd have to think laterally to make it interesting and ended up creating some of the earliest data graphics. Her bosses thought they were so good they became a template for the way they did the news. 'But it was exhausting. I was always starting about 30 per cent behind the ones – usually young, posh, white men – who were given the juicy stories. To make mine sing I had to think long and hard. Black women and Asian women like me always have to be twice as good and put in three times as much effort. My advice is to find pathways that give you the edge – it's been my mantra.'

She talked about the cultural pressure she'd always felt to 'be collegiate, not to draw attention to myself' as an Asian woman. Most of her life has been spent behind the camera, in the edit suite. But as she approaches sixty, she is finally turning up the volume on herself and her life; she now posts regularly on LinkedIn. 'I share my experiences and my views, I have a lot to offer, I have been in my profession for thirty years. I found it hard to find my voice; at first it felt very uncomfortable to speak out, but by sharing my inner narrative, what I really think, I am getting great traction. More than I could have dared to believe.' At fifty-eight Lalita is finally blowing her own trumpet, putting herself out there. The result? A rejuvenated career as a thought-leader in the digital space. She is thrilled by the impact she is having and the invitations to speak she now receives, but 'along with the excitement and the pleasure I also feel angry: angry at the conditioning that kept me silent for so long, at the freedom and power I could have enjoyed earlier'.

Lalita's shift into her Queenager power – like the stories of so many women at this point – emerged out of loss. Her husband died suddenly just before he was fifty. Lalita was at home with her son who had a bad foot when she got a call from her husband's work saying he had keeled over and collapsed. 'A police car arrived at my door to whizz me to the hospital. He'd had a huge heart attack – we had no idea, he was fit as a flea, rode his bike everywhere, never smoked. He was forty-nine. Our children were fifteen and seventeen. They tried to resuscitate him for an hour but it was no good. He was dead.'

His death was so sudden Lalita had an out-of-body experience. 'I heard wailing, screaming – I didn't realise it was me.' For three days she couldn't do anything. Then she pulled herself together 'for my kids. I looked after them. I went back to work to pay the bills. It was a dark, tough time.'

But as I hear so often from many Queenagers, that forged-in-fire moment, when her old life as she'd known it came to an end, also turned out, eventually, to be a liberation. Until that point Lalita had seen herself primarily as a wife and mother. But she now felt she could finally create her own identity, the roles she chose. 'I feel these are my golden years, that I am in my prime. I am using my fifties to set myself up for my sixties, which I know are going to be my best yet.'

Like me, Lalita has learnt how important it is to use and voice all the experience and wisdom we have as women in our Queenager years. 'The world really needs it. And by creating a strong brand for myself now I feel I can future-proof myself to be a consultant, to go on being relevant into my sixties and seventies.' Lalita's strong suit is technology. She wants other Queenagers to upskill themselves, particularly around AI, so that they can go on being relevant and speak up. 'After all, if not now – when? No one will do it for you. You need to have the confidence to realise how much you have to offer. I've learnt to advocate for myself both behind the scenes and in the open. And that means I can give back and open up opportunities for other women. I just wish I had known this before. That is why I am speaking up now.'

Lalita is increasingly mentoring younger diverse founders. 'I draw such energy from these incredible, purposeful, inspiring young people. I can open doors for them. Tell them how it was for me. Connect them to people I know – point them in the right direction.' She calls this the 'sweet time', when women of experience can help the next generation. This chimes massively with what we found in our research about Queenagers wanting to give back, to pass on their hard-earned wisdom to the women coming up behind.

Personally, Lalita is also in a good place. 'After my husband died I realised it was pointless to save things for best; we had all these crystal glasses and smart clothes that we'd been saving and then he died, having never used any of them. So I went out and spent some money on myself – I'd started a business on the side which was doing well. I bought nice clothes and handbags. I had some treatments. I went on holidays. I started online dating and now have a lovely partner.' I admire the way Lalita has invested in herself to make the most of her new chapter. 'I chose joy, not despair. It is a choice, you know, however dark the times.' I love her story because it is so hopeful. She told me how her mother had grown up in the deserts of Rajasthan, in a family so poor that often there was no milk and when there was milk it was given to her brothers. Lalita's mother went to school but got into trouble with her teachers for having to write all her subject lessons in one notebook, which was all she could afford. For that she was punished by having to stand outside in the midday sun. 'My mum is so proud to see what I have become,' Lalita says. 'She worked so hard to escape the poverty of her beginnings, so that I could have a good life.' She is living proof of the power of progress. Of the magic of Queenager becoming but also of how much life for women has changed for the better around the globe.

These are Lalita's ten tips for success:

1. Always be kind to yourself.
2. Build networks – professional, special interests and fun.
3. Find your North Star – mine was technology.
4. Read longform and keep a journal.
5. Meet people in real life.
6. Look after yourself – investing in your youth will keep you looking good as you grow old.
7. Eat well and mindfully – enjoy every bite.
8. Take up new hobbies – it keeps you young.
9. Be generous and the universe smiles at you.
10. Find opportunities to give back – volunteer!

I love Lalita's calm, unflappable manner and her determined optimism; she is living proof that there is so much more to come.

Secret: The clearing of a space in midlife, however painful at the time, can reap us a huge benefit in the end.

Making the decision to quit

I always felt lucky to know what it was I wanted to do. I left university and became a journalist, working first for the deeply unglamorous *Tank World* and *Container Management* magazines, writing about cranes and containers at international ports (the highlight was being allowed to drive a huge spreader, a kind of crane that lifts and stacks 40-metre containers – I felt like a kid in a Tonka truck). The office was next to a motorway; if we saw a tank container we'd written about driving along we'd yell. Exciting, huh?

Others are equally purpose-driven from the start. Take Lizzie, who had wanted to work for the NHS since she was four and had cardiac surgery to fill a hole in her heart; when she woke up after the operation a 'lovely nurse helped me eat my banana custard, and I've wanted to be her ever since. I even announced as much to my mum as we drove home from hospital.'

Yet even those of us who love our jobs can need a change after a couple of decades. Sometimes we've done everything we can do, other times the world, or we, have changed and it just doesn't fit us anymore. Increasingly, technology might mean the job we used to do doesn't exist.

It's hard being whacked from a job you love, but it can also be agony to leave somewhere out of choice because it's just not working for you anymore. I love Lizzie's story because it speaks so much to that growing sense of disenchantment, the tussle between what you thought you wanted and the reality; and the courage it takes to make a change. Particularly when you are living your childhood dream and it is your life.

When I was whacked it was awful – but with the benefit of hindsight I am grateful; because I don't think I would have had the courage to walk away myself, even though I knew I was stale and needed a change, and because I am now so much happier. Knowing that I wouldn't have been brave enough to jump makes me even more full of admiration for those who make the first move, who realise they need to leave and have the gumption to do so – particularly when, like Lizzie, they walk away from a phalanx of friends, a whole tribe who have made the job worthwhile, and a lifelong vocation.

Lizzie had worked in the NHS as a nurse for twenty-two years, almost as long as my stint at the paper. When she finally resigned she shed heavy tears, her team hugged her, but 'my heart felt bruised'. She had graduated as a degree-level nurse, then worked in the emergency department as a nurse practitioner through two pregnancies. Being faced with life-and-death situations really used to get her adrenaline pumping and she says that even after two decades she 'never lost the thrill I felt when running to the resuscitation room after the red phone rang warning of an incoming emergency. My mind would light up thinking about what was coming, what would we need to do, how would we do it, could we save the patient?' It was exhilarating to save someone who without you might not have made it, but for all the times when it went well there were others when she was left defeated. She said that she is still haunted by the people who didn't make it. 'Seeing the suffering of the families often broke me. But then I'd look at younger members of the team struggling to cope and I knew how much I had learnt about trauma.'

Of course, in such intense jobs it is the camaraderie that gets you through, the tribe of close colleagues who always have your back as you have theirs. Nursing, like journalism, involves long, awkward hours and compromises on how much you see your family. Your team are your world. 'It was my friends who kept me in nursing so long. The hospital is like my second home.'

But as the years rolled on – Lizzie was now forty-seven – she said it became harder and harder to keep going. 'Those days I just felt permanently exhausted. Take my last shift – I had three patients on the go: I'd put a plaster cast on a boy's broken arm and sent him to a ward to await his operation; another patient was on a drip with a septic wound, while the third was an old lady with a head wound.' Lizzie explained that the ward was so busy all the time she didn't even have five minutes to visit the toilet, let alone eat a meal. In her time as a nurse the work volume increased exponentially while the financial rewards just decreased.

'The price I paid for doing this job increasingly felt too high. It was not just money. It was the antisocial hours, the life-and-death responsibility, the inability to solve the problems.' She said she had seen an explosion in self-harm and mental health services that were completely overstretched. 'My heart broke for my patients but there was only so much help we could give them. I was in that triple lock of feeling like I was failing as a mother, nurse *and* daughter.' That sense of failing on all fronts was exacerbated by the antisocial hours Lizzie worked; she was always on shift when her family and friends were off and vice versa. When her kids were small the upside of doing those hours was that her husband could cover the childcare and she got paid extra. 'But when the kids were bigger the trade-off just wasn't worth it.' Lizzie sounded burnt-out; she said she often felt 'spent' emotionally and physically after a 'killer shift'. 'The stress could drown me and, just as the mum guilt grew, the nurse guilt also grew. I didn't feel like I was doing or offering the best of me wherever I was.'

Lizzie reluctantly came to realise that, in her mid-forties, she could not go on, that for her own well-being and sanity, and for her family, she needed to do something more wholesome and restorative. 'Patching people together again as an emergency nurse was too narrow. I realised that for the rest of my career I wanted to make people really feel better in all aspects of their lives, to look after them more holistically, so they could achieve true and sustainable wellness.'

She accepted a job in a doctor's surgery where she would be the first line of contact for all their patients. She'd work better hours, for better pay – and it would be far less draining.

'What I want is to be able to make things better for my patients, like those nurses did for me when I was four. It is such a relief to finally stop.'

Lizzie was right. As we age the stress that once made us feel alive, pumped with adrenaline, raring to go, can stop having that effect. Maybe we've just done it too much, or maybe that life suited us then – or helped us to block out our own problems with busyness for a while – but then it doesn't serve us anymore. Many Queenagers get to a point where they realise it is time to take all their experience and skills and use them in a different way. Often we can redeploy to improve our own lives, take a bit more care of ourselves rather than putting everybody else's needs first. I hear this so often, but Lizzie's case is such a good exemplar. So, if that feels familiar, like the job you loved is no longer serving *your* needs, think about a change … you matter too. You can take your experience and deploy it to find a new version of you. Yes, it feels daunting but that will pass. Try to feel not just scared but excited; after all, a whole new chapter awaits.

Secret: What works for us when we are young doesn't necessarily go on serving us as we get older. That's okay. It's not a sign of failure to want a change of direction or if something you loved no longer lights your fire. Make a change, embrace it. It might just be the best thing you ever did.

The 'dream' job

I talk about 'Queenagers' because there is something adolescent about this period of young-oldness, shifting into the beginning of the second half of our lives. We are starting a new phase, some of us are a bit hormonal (just like teenagers) and we are feeling the growing pains of transition; that pupa stage where we know what we don't want, or can't do anymore, but haven't quite sussed what comes next. Chip Conley, the American modern elder, calls midlife not a crisis but a chrysalis. He is right. This time is all a big transition from what we were to what we might become.

I wanted to capture something of the possibility of this point, the optimism amid the fear of the unknown. In our research what came across very clearly from the women was that there was an urgency, a sense of 'this is *my* time, I've been looking after everyone else for thirty years, this is when I finally get to be me!' And also a very clear drumbeat of 'if not now, when?' – that sense that we still have our health and our drive but who knows how much longer it will last. That 'Time's wingèd chariot [is] hurrying near', as the poet Andrew Marvell put it.

What goes along with that urgency to get on with it is often a determination to pursue the path less travelled, the part of ourselves that got away, that got lost while life had other plans for us; families, earning a living – normal stuff. But for me the huge promise of this moment is, with many of our earlier boxes ticked, we finally get a chance to go back to what *we* want to do. By the time we hit fiftyish, we have ticked off everything that our parents or society told us we *should* be doing and got through that, successfully or not. Weirdly, at this point it kind of doesn't matter; if it was successful it is still done, and if it wasn't that great, it is still over and also done. Either way it is time to ring in the new.

What I have seen repeatedly in groups, on retreats, in conversations, in the audiences of the many talks I have given, is this hunger in the women I meet to scratch that itch, do the thing they always really wanted to do – before it is too late. And the whole point of this book is to make you, dear reader, realise that that applies to you too; that it's not too late, you are not too old, that there is still much more to come, however bleak things may have seemed.

For me that itch is to write books. I have always been a writer. When I was a little girl I wrote poems; I had a special book decorated with pictures of flowers into which I would transcribe them, religiously. I read English Literature at university because I wanted to be an author – although, truth be told, the experience put me off trying to write my own book for thirty years. Journalism, history's first draft – the quickness of it, the 'write it and it's done, tomorrow's chip paper' – seemed easier. I loved the immediacy of hackery, the knowing, the reporting, the poking about and asking questions, the sense of telling a story that mattered and getting it out into the world in real time.

Real writing, books, novels … that gave me the fear. The pressure of all that literary criticism I'd read; the impossibility of expressing anything new, anything that might be worth saying. I'm still not immune. I went back to my old college in Oxford to see my daughter who is studying there now (English, just like me – yes, I am *super*-proud). 'How's the book going?' she asked me over lunch. I mumbled something. She got all English studenty on me: 'What are you really trying to say? What is it going to be memorable for? What will people quote?' She is naturally forensic and was trying to be nice, but her questions floored me. The doubt and uncertainty set in. I didn't write a word for about a month afterwards; the self-doubt became crippling.

So I do understand. W. B. Yeats was right when he wrote, 'tread softly because you tread on my dreams'. Dreams are fragile. Having the courage to sit with a blank piece of paper and express ourselves is hard and hard-won. It's why some of my favourite stories of midlife re-creation and inspiration are those of women who have done just that. Found the confidence to speak up, found their voice. That is so hard to do!

For some it is raising a family which stops them pursuing their dreams. Others are held back by the limiting beliefs society puts on them. That's why I love this story, from Julie Owen Moylan, so much. She reached out to me when I first started Noon and she had me with the very beginning of the e-mail she wrote when she described how every time she visited a bookshop she would 'find the place on the shelf where if I were to write a book you might find it and I would make a space for it. Leaving a tiny gap that one day might be filled with my book became a good-luck charm, it was a way of showing myself that my dreams of being a writer were not dead.'

I love the way we keep those secret bits of ourselves alive, that inner ambition burning even if it is only manifested through small, clandestine acts. Julie explained that her dreams weren't technically alive 'because she never did anything active about them', but she still burnt to be a writer and used to scribble little stories on notepads all the time.

So why didn't she pursue her dream earlier? Julie explains that the large, soulless educational establishment she attended was 'designed to churn out an army of shorthand typists and manual workers. We didn't have a sixth form. We had no need of it. There was no career marked "writer" that I was aware of.'

Her grandmother had been a cleaner and her dearest wish was that Julie's mother wouldn't have to clean up after other people. 'My mother worked in factories before she married and her wish was that I would work in an office. We had limited ambitions because we didn't know there were other possibilities for people who lived in council houses.'

Julie describes how on careers day she stood in a long line of bored kids waiting to be granted an audience with the physics teacher who moonlighted as careers adviser. She was due to leave school that summer but had no idea what she wanted to do. 'I didn't know how to say, "I want to be a writer"; there wasn't anyone I could say it to. As the line shuffled along, the girl in front of me said she wanted to be a hairdresser. It sounded creative to me, like the closest I was going to get to working in the arts, so when it was my turn I said the same thing and took an application form for the local tech college. And that was it.'

She describes how for 'the longest time I carried around a committee in my head of people who ran my life. They had "useful" messages to keep me in line. "Helpful" phrases like "Who do you think you are?" and "You're too old to try." I don't know exactly when this committee moved in, but when I turned fifty years old I knew I really wanted them to move out. The eviction process was hard because it involved risk and fear. Fear of failing. Fear of looking stupid. Fear of shattering my dreams because if you don't try, then you can't fail and you can still believe that it could happen. Battling myself for the right to try was the first step in a ten-year journey to become an author.'

For Julie's fiftieth birthday she gave herself the gift of a part-time master's in creative writing. It was held over two evenings a week for the best part of a year, with a further six months to submit a dissertation. She would cover short stories and novel writing in a small group of varying ages and abilities. Julie drank it up. 'I read *everything* on the reading list. I once flew back from a holiday in New York, landed and still made the evening seminar. That's how much I wanted to learn. By the time I'd completed my master's degree I was pretty good at constructing short stories. They arrived fully formed most of the time and, on one glorious day, I had two submissions accepted for publication in different magazines.'

The exhilaration of finally being a writer, of having given herself permission to write and now reaping the rewards, was heady. 'When my tutor marked my dissertation, he declared the 10,000 words of a novel I'd submitted as publishable quality and I was ecstatic, believing it was just a matter of time before I completed my debut novel and the literary world fell at my feet.' It wasn't that easy. Julie failed time and again to get a literary agent, the people who act as the gatekeepers of the publishing world. There are many literary agents, mostly based in London, and they are inundated with submissions. It's a long process waiting for responses and often they never arrive. 'My first novel got seventy rejections and I was crushed. My old committee popped back up to tell me they had been right all along. I was too old … not good enough … the dream was over.'

Except it wasn't over. She enrolled on an online novel-writing course which promised professional feedback and introductions to agents. Tentatively she wrote the opening scene of her idea for a novel and put it online for the rest of the group to critique. 'The absolute horror of that is not to be underestimated and I couldn't think of one single idea, but then an opening line drifted into my mind and I wrote, "The day the box arrived, my mother thought she was Jesus." That line turned into the opening chapters and, with support and feedback from my tutor, it became the first draft of my novel.'

It was a dark November day many months later when Julie checked her e-mail and saw to her surprise that several literary agents had got in touch to say they loved the opening and wanted to read more. Over the next two weeks she met with some of the biggest names in publishing and by Christmas she'd signed with an agent. 'In the end I signed a two-book deal and my debut novel, *That Green Eyed Girl*, is now in the shops. I still go into bookshops and make a space for my book. The difference this time is it's there. You're never too old. Never give up on your dreams.'

I love this story, and I love Julie. When I e-mailed her to ask if she'd mind me using her in this book she said, 'Of course. *That Green Eyed Girl* has been successful and my second novel, *73 Dove Street*, is also published. I've also signed a contract for two more, so it has very much worked out for me. I really hope your book encourages other Queenagers to go for it!' So do I.

Secret: We all start off with a dream – when we hit about fifty we realise that if that dream is ever going to materialise then we need to get on with it, that time is running out. So what was your dream? What did young you really want to be before life got in the way? … Now's the time!

The mature student

Some disabilities are visible. Others are not. In our lifetime we have seen massive shifts in understanding around mental health and disorders such as ADHD and dyslexia. For women particularly, who are often socially skilled so can 'mask' their symptoms, diagnoses of these conditions are rocketing – in the last number of years in the UK there has been an exponential increase in adults with ADHD largely because it is better recognised. One friend recounted how when she took her daughter to the doctor and he went through the symptoms – impulsiveness, disorganisation, poor time management skills, difficulty focusing and restlessness – my pal realised that she had all the symptoms too. She's started taking medication and says for the first time in her life it's as if all the distractions in her brain have been switched off and she can concentrate.

When I was at school, children displaying these symptoms were just branded troublesome, or stupid; discarded because the standard model didn't fit the way they learnt or behaved. Many left school without any formal qualifications. In my experience, dyslexics in particular tend to be highly intelligent, with a different take on the world, and are some of the brightest people I've ever met (and the list of entrepreneurs in this category is endless, from Jamie Oliver to Richard Branson).

One of my jobs at the *Sunday Times* was to edit the genius journalist A. A. Gill. He was so dyslexic that he couldn't write his own copy, he dictated it. When it arrived, it would be a stream of consciousness with no punctuation, the words running together. If it was late for a deadline – say, election coverage where he had been out sketching a particular politician on the stump, filing as the paper was going to press – it would be terrifying. I'd have a whole page of the newspaper waiting for his article and what would arrive would look like unpublishable nonsense. But then I would take a deep breath, sit and go through it slowly, working out by sounding the words aloud phonetically what they were supposed to be; things like changing 'melon collie' to 'melancholy'. Putting in commas and sentences and capital letters. And suddenly it would spring to life. Shining like a diamond. The best writing in the paper, even though he couldn't 'write'. It was a lesson never to judge anything superficially.

I always think of A. A. Gill when I talk to Molly. She is a pin-up for midlife transformation. She left school at sixteen with no qualifications. Her neurodiversity and dyslexia were so severe that school was a washout for her. She carries deep shame as a result. So much so that, even at fifty, talking about it can bring her to tears. She shouldn't be ashamed. She is highly intelligent. When I used to write a weekly column, I would try out my lines on her before I put fingers to keyboard. She always had something germane to contribute, usually something I hadn't thought of. Years of being a personal fitness trainer led her to qualifying to teach Pilates. In terms of body and mind I have never met anyone so fascinated by how the brain works, or so intuitively in touch with what her clients need. So when she said she wanted to go and do a neuroscience master's degree at the beginning of lockdown and would I help her apply, I said a big yes. And lo and behold she was accepted on the Neuroscience MSc programme at King's College London, where she proceeded to smash it and get a 2:1 – with the help of AI technology which turns speech into writing (and a scribe when she needed it).

I see many women in our Noon community going back to university to study at fifty. One was sick of her career as a diplomat and went back to retrain as a doctor (working on the wards during Covid – now *that's* fulfilling a vocation). Another went back to study sociology, another literature. Many Queenagers seem to be qualifying as counsellors or coaches. But given Molly's history of failure with academia I wondered what had given her the confidence to go to university for the first time at fifty. 'Something is changing for me at this point in my life. Things are possible which weren't before. There's always been a crazy ambition in me and it is the support of other wonderful, clever women in my life – friends and clients – who made me feel that with their help I could pull this off.'

Her journey was boosted by the fact that Molly's daughter also has ADHD. 'I suppose watching her struggle and thinking about how my neurodiversity has affected my whole life made me want to understand more about what was going on inside my head.'

Of course, having the piece of paper hasn't wiped away all those years of self-doubt. 'I hoped that having a degree would erase all those negative feelings, that all that bad self-worth would vanish. But life isn't like that. My "I'm not enough" complex is still alive and kicking, it is rooted in my brain, linked to the ADHD and the dyslexia. It's chemical, elemental in me that my mind is always jumping from one thing to another – it's like having sixteen television channels inside my head all blaring at once. There is always a serial narrative running, there is no peace.' Molly explains that when her mind wanders, which it does constantly, most of the time it goes into dark areas, ruminating over anxiety, stress and worry, which sends her onto emotional rollercoasters.

But the worst side of ADHD is how hard it makes it to regulate emotions. 'I would feel very sad, literally be unable to stop myself crying if I was being told off by a teacher, or in a meeting with a boss. And then I would be very mouthy and loud and pretend I didn't care in order to survive.'

Molly says that tough front was also put on because of the British stiff upper lip and embarrassment around emotion. 'My way was *not* the normal way. It left me so humiliated, my self-esteem in the dust. And school was the worst. I didn't engage, it was just one shameful experience after another.'

Molly internalised all the emotional dysregulation. 'You are convinced you are not good enough, that you can't do anything because you can't concentrate, can't write. I was made to feel so stupid. I would try so hard, feel so hurt, and then get angry and defensive.'

She learnt to wear a mask. To relate from a peripheral perspective to hide what she was feeling. 'I have worked hard on my physical beauty. [Molly has a boob job and a body that most 20-year-olds would envy thanks to three decades of daily Pilates.] But it is a screen to hide my vulnerability, I am a terrible people pleaser, co-dependent. Along with getting my master's I also found the courage to leave my marriage in my forties. A liberation.'

What Molly is describing is the upside of the midlife collision – the strength to walk away from a bad marriage, the courage to put aside all her negative feelings about education and come out with a master's in neuroscience. A true-life transformation. Of course, that shift doesn't come without pain. It is staggering how often we are thrown back into our deepest fears, those dark bits of ourselves. But learning to sit with them, accept them, realise they will always be there but they don't have to stop us moving forward if we don't let them – that is the midlife work.

These days Molly sees her neurodiversity as simultaneously her cross to bear and her superpower. 'It's *because* of all of it that I am deeply kind and empathetic. I want to care for people.' For a couple of decades Molly worked as a nanny and looked after rejected teenagers in the care system. 'I can relate to other people who are in pain; the ADHD gives me another emotional gear. I have a deep capacity for friendship; I am surrounded by people who love me – I am the fun, the party, the light. My life is about relationships and bringing joy to those around me.'

There is another upside to ADHD, she has discovered. As well as fracturing the attention span, it also gives sufferers the capacity to enter into a hyper-focused state. Molly describes this as, 'To truly be in joy. To be totally in flow for a really long time. I find that when I am doing something that I really love – styling people, finding them exactly the right clothes to suit them, their life and their body, or working as a coach – I am super-focused, I can keep going for hours, I just never want to stop.' She has just used her master's to qualify as a life coach and says, 'I enter that wonderful flow state when I am working with clients too, everything comes together. I also see that in my daughter; she is becoming a hairdresser and she can just do it for hours. It is like our superpower.'

Secret: Often our biggest flaw can become our shining light. There is joy in resilience, in winning through. In loving ourselves enough to be sympathetic to our inner trauma but not to let it defeat us.

Pivot into purpose

My granny always used to say, 'Darling, no job will *ever* love you back.' It was her way of intimating that I was working too hard, overcommitted. I remembered her words when I was chairing an International Women's Day panel and a young woman in the audience asked how many hours a week the members of the panel worked on average; she said she was ambitious and wanted to do well in her career, but she didn't want it to take over her life. She had young kids. What she was after was an honest answer about what it was going to take to make it to the top.

It was a tricky moment. On the panel next to me were two other female founders, the head of a travel company (a man) and the head of HR of a huge corporate. The man said he worked at least seventy hours a week. The two founders admitted to being workaholics, saying they did at least seventy hours and maybe more. And then it came to me. I said that if you totted up the hours I spent doing stuff for my community of women, or thinking about them, or writing, it was probably a large number. But the bigger point was about how it made me feel. When I was a newspaper executive and always on someone else's time and dollar, I felt constantly stressed; chivvied, hustled, made to feel bad if I was five or ten minutes late in the morning even if I was going to work till midnight that night. Usually I was late not because I was lazy or inefficient but because I'd done a whole second shift before I got to the damn office. A typical morning would involve preparing two packed lunches, retrieving swimming or gym kit from the bottom of a wash basket, making a World Book Day costume, or finishing some other kind of crucial school project, finding and doing the homework, breaking up a fight or being a counsellor over some emotional drama – not to mention getting myself dressed and arriving in the office with a list of ideas for the next day's paper.

I used to look enviously at the men with stay-at-home wives who had nothing to do before work except, maybe, trot along to the gym, or read the papers over a relaxed cup of coffee. Of course, once I got to work, the mayhem would truly start: my entire day would be mapped out for me – meetings I had to attend, which would land in my diary without consultation; always I was at the beck and call of a host of senior men. I'd often have to spend hours shooting the breeze with my boss, chatting about his weekend or the state of the world, while internally I was chafing, knowing every minute I sat with him meant having to work later and possibly missing bedtime. I always felt like I wasn't doing enough, being enough, wasn't enough! That however much I did, however hard I drove myself, I was short-changing someone. And the reality? I sort of was.

These days, however, although I work hard, I *love* what I do. And, best of all, I am in charge of my time. If I want to stop, I stop. At noon every day I go and swim in the pond. I turn off my phone. I look at the sun through the leaves and the parakeets screeching and tweeting in the trees. I don't have to be reachable at all times; I am the boss. Sometimes I work late, or am fiddling around on social media when my husband is going to sleep (he *hates* that). Some evenings I do events with my Queenagers, or I even take them off to foreign countries for adventures, or run retreats, but it doesn't feel like work – it feels like fun. I love it all; it fills me with joy, with a sense of achievement, with purpose. I often get e-mails saying how much something I have written or done has helped someone or made them feel better about themselves. That gives me a warm glow inside. In fact, I am fired up by purpose and passion; we really are changing the world, one Queenager at a time.

So that is a long way of saying that working seventy hours a week on a passion project that is all yours is totally different from working for a psycho in a huge organisation, however status-ful or well paid. If you work for someone else, you can be fired at any moment. I remember a wise woman saying to me: 'Your true capital is everything you would still have if you lost your job title and salary tomorrow.' Yes, read that again. It's true. So make sure you are enriching your wider networks.

What saved me after being made redundant was all the work I had done as chair of Women in Journalism and the huge network I had there, the research, the thinking. When the job stopped, WIJ was still there. It was a lifeline. So think about that in terms of your own life. Are you creating a safety net? Are you making connections outside your immediate employer, into the wider industry? Are you thinking about what comes next, what you would do? Do you have a passion project or a side hustle? If not, maybe start thinking about what that could look like for you because no organisation is ever loyal, whatever they may say. At some point you will become dispensable, and what will you do then?

Also, if you work for yourself then it is all yours, your e-mail list, your money, your clients. If you work with someone you don't like, it's only for a day or so and they are paying you enough to make it worthwhile. And for me the difference is that sense of purpose, of agency, of doing something I love and that feels worthwhile – and that *I choose*. I don't *have* to do what my boss says. Or think in the way that he does, or squish my own thoughts and world-view to accommodate someone else's – which I did for *far* too long. I feel buoyant and full of purpose; I love paddling my own canoe and feeling like I am making the world a better place. Sure, 'Freedom has no sponsor', as a surfer I met in Puerto Escondido in Mexico once told me. But it also has no boss. Yippee.

And that midlife pivot into purpose is common for women at this point. We've called it 'The Revolt'. It also helps compensate for what we feel we have lost. Let's take Sue. She was editor for thirty years of a huge weekly magazine that you will definitely have read. She was at the top of her game, and then suddenly she wasn't. With no explanation she was out.

Her job had absorbed her every waking hour and then it ended, abruptly. Unable to process the turmoil of difficult emotions that overwhelmed her, Sue succumbed first to chronic anxiety and then panic attacks. 'I was consumed by a nameless terror and sense of dread, suddenly unable to function as a normal human being. I rapidly became a prisoner in my own home.'

During the day, her friends and family rallied round but night-time was difficult. For weeks she couldn't sleep despite trying everything from meditation to listening to the radio and pacing around her house. 'My heart pounded in panic, blood raced through my veins, and the tangle of thoughts endlessly tumbled round in my head. At those times – when things were at their darkest – I would lie with my phone on the bedside table next to me, the Samaritans number on the screen, primed and ready for me simply to press the green button. I realised then how important it was to know that – at whatever time of day or night (and, let's face it, things often seem much worse in the dead of night) – there was someone I could speak to, someone who would simply be there.' Sue never actually called the Samaritans but she didn't forget how reassured she had felt by knowing that she could.

I felt such empathy with Sue's story. That sense of being unmoored, in freefall, untethered from all life's usual landmarks, was so familiar to me. Sudden transitions shake us to our foundations, evoke high levels of anxiety even in those of us who thought we were admirably grounded and stable. And, as we so often see in Queenagers, Sue was hit by the midlife maelstrom. Just over a year after she was made redundant, Sue's beloved mother died. It was another bitter blow.

'That terrible year ended with my mum's funeral. Her health had been deteriorating for several months, and her death brought another shocking – and grief-filled – full stop in my life. I started to wonder how I might fill the gap left by my mother and my work tribe; I also missed the stories that had been shared with me when I was an editor. Most of all I wanted a sense of purpose again.'

Sue told me that for over a year she'd felt like flotsam, tossed around on a sea of emotions as she struggled to sort her life out and support her mother. Sue realised she needed to find a new outlet for herself. That was when she remembered the Samaritans and suddenly thought that working for them might give her back the purpose she craved. She found a branch close to her home through Google and went along to an information evening.

She liked what she found so much that she signed up, attended a full day of workshops, got the relevant security/criminal checks and was selected for the training course – ten three-hour modules spread over three months, each of them compulsory. Once out of the classroom, she did twenty three-hour shifts alongside mentors, spread over four months. And then, finally, she 'flew solo' – carrying out shifts without a mentor (but always at the branch, with at least one other trained listening volunteer on duty). Four more training modules later she 'achieved my number – a unique group of digits showing that you are now a fully fledged Samaritans listening volunteer. The whole process takes the best part of a year, and the sense of pride at achieving your number is considerable.'

The joy of learning a new skill was crucial to Sue's new sense of purpose and satisfaction. As an editor she'd been expected to think on her feet, stay calm in a crisis, have an opinion on everything and find instant solutions. At the Samaritans she learnt to 'actively listen' to really hear what the caller is saying, to understand, support and empathise with their distress, to emotionally 'hold' them while they unburden. She learnt how to say the right things, give 'verbal cuddles', allow silence and resist the temptation to interrupt, judge, or offer advice or solutions. Sue admits that if anyone had told her four years ago that her future would involve becoming a Samaritan she would have laughed. But she says that learning to help people 'go towards the pain', listening to them express their feelings and deepest fears without recoiling at unpleasant or shocking revelations, has been an incredible adventure and privilege.

Sue is adamant that she gains as much from helping her callers as they do from her calm and responsive listening. Much of what she hears is harrowing. Take, for instance, her caller Pauline, who had recently lost her husband, who spoke about her concerns for her adult son whose mental health issues meant that he will never lead an independent life. 'At the end of the call Pauline said, "I never asked your name – what is it?" Before I could reply, she said, "No, it's okay. I'm going to call you Angel, because you've been an angel to me tonight." She couldn't have made me happier if she'd presented me with a Nobel Prize.'

Sue's story so perfectly expresses how we can use our own life reversals to shift into a new purposeful phase of giving back and, by doing so, heal not only ourselves but others, too. That has to be the ultimate Queenager win-win.

Secret: Moving into purpose, working for a cause bigger than yourself which allows you to give something positive back, is a great healer.

Sistering – we rise together

When you look at other women, what goes through your mind? Do you look at them as your sisters, with love, with admiration for their essence? Or do you judge, measuring yourself against them? I have been thinking more about the deep rifts in sisterhood, the ways we have been taught to judge and distrust each other as women. In essence this is 'divide and rule', that old colonial favourite of making different tribes of the conquered fight each other, to distract them from uniting against the true aggressor. If women are divided from each other, taught to distrust and judge each other, we won't band together and use our collective power to change our lot. This is one of the parts of our conditioning that is most crucial to unpick. It is one of the reasons I feel so passionate about the supportive Queenager community we have created at Noon.

Recently I attended a sistering workshop run by Clare Dubois, the founder of TreeSisters. Clare is one of the most impressive, powerful women I have ever met. When I first left my big job, she helped me hugely. We spoke on Zoom and I told her that, despite spending twenty-five years as a writer and a columnist, I was having real trouble expressing myself now that I was trying to write from the heart in my own voice rather than that of my old paper. At that point, I burst into tears. Quite embarrassing, as she is an icon who has addressed crowds of tens of thousands of people at huge festivals on the subject of climate change and replanting trees to save the planet, and there was me, a snivelling whacked journalist, in my bedroom, sobbing because I was finding it hard to write what I felt. But I shouldn't have worried. The tears forged a strong connection between us; she leant into my vulnerability and stretched out a helping hand.

'Aah,' she said. 'It's not a weakness in you. It is hard. True expression of the feminine always comes with pain. With constriction of the throat – the voice chakra. Like all our internal programming it is trying to protect us from what will happen if we speak out. Like an unconscious mechanism stopping us from putting ourselves in danger. As a woman historically and in many parts of the world still today, it is risky to speak up, to speak truth, particularly to power. The emergent female voice is born through tears, through fear, through pain. Just accept the pain comes with the territory – and the fear – and just write it anyway. It will get easier the more you do it.'

It was one of the best pieces of advice I've ever been given. Up there with change is difficult. Because it is true; it is something I pass on to other women when they are also struggling to express themselves, or scared of the consequences. It comes from hundreds of years of women being told to be seen and not heard. Of the punishment for women who didn't obey their husbands or the codes of their society being death. This is not so long ago. Speaking out as a woman is still a death sentence in parts of the world today. Think of brave Malala who spoke out for the right for girls to be educated in Pakistan and was shot in the head for her pains. Or the girls in Afghanistan who aren't allowed to go to school and the women there banned from parks or going to the hairdresser's by a misogynist regime. Or the women and girls of Iran killed for speaking out against compulsory Islamic dress.

At the sistering workshop, Clare led sixty women outside to sit under a majestic oak tree. We settled in the grass among the roots. She talked about the historical persecution of women, how for several centuries in Europe women were burnt as witches, regularly. Thousands of women between the Middle Ages and the Victorian era were accused of witchcraft. Often their offences were as anodyne as talking to another woman or women (this was denounced as 'plotting'); or being a widow (with a handsome fortune). Any kind of female independence from men was seen as a witchy threat; 'the safest thing for a woman to do was to shackle herself to a man and shun her sisters if she didn't want to be killed,' explained Clare. Of course, this was all sanctioned and often arranged by the official Church after the 'witches' had been identified by people in their immediate communities, who often held a grudge against them. Most often it was single women, widows, midwives, those who ministered to other women in the old ways, those who challenged the patriarchal norms, who were singled out. We women know that when we are with other women we become in sync, whether that's something as basic as our periods happening at the same time, or having an intuitive sense of when a sister we love is in trouble. It was precisely that sisterly bond that the witch trials set out to destroy.

'We women feel everything,' said Clare. 'Empathy and sensitivity to each other are wired into the female body. But it's as if those parts of our nature have been bound and gagged by memory of the huge witch trauma, even though it is not in our generation. The legacy of the witch trials and burnings is like a cosmic car crash for female relations; because of the witch experience it is hard-wired into us to be suspicious of other women, to judge them, to shun them for our own safety.'

We may not usually associate our quickness to judge other women with witches – but we have been so programmed to give our sisters the once-over (and not always kindly) that we do it unconsciously. Don't believe me? Just think about walking down a street. We women look at other women's bodies or outfits or behaviours and judge and critique them.

To allow us all to see what is getting in the way of us just being loving and supportive to each other, Clare set us a series of tasks. First, we had to choose a partner at random and sit opposite them, gazing into their eyes. One of the pair had to just gaze at the other one with total love and acceptance, while the other kept up a monologue for two minutes of how that felt. I found the gazing with love interesting. Quietening the way our brains can leap into critique, intentionally, was tricky to start with – but by my third partner it had got much easier; any muscle strengthens with use. It was a revelation to gaze on another woman with total love and adoration, thinking how beautiful her hair or eyes were. The gentleness of her gaze, the vulnerability in her face.

But being the recipient of the gaze was unsettling. I felt hot and uncomfortable under scrutiny. I wanted to look away as the intimacy of holding such intense eye contact with a stranger was hard. But the process acted as a kind of unpeeling. In one of the exercises, rather than saying how we felt, we had to say what we wanted to let go of. That is pretty deep and fundamental stuff; and what comes out isn't necessarily what we think. Some of our bad habits, when it comes down to it, we don't want to shed. Other stuff we want to jettison is really profound and painful. I cried through most of that session; and my tears were met by compassion and understanding from a sister I had only just met. It felt good to be met with so much love and trust. It made me see how often we don't approach other women with those feelings. How we can be competitive or resentful, jealous or snooty and undermining; we don't mean to be, it's just what, on a deep and unconscious level, we've been taught.

Catching that conditioning as it plays out, seeing it in ourselves and understanding it, means we can change. It's like finally seeing the matrix that we live within. Which means we can challenge it. Do something different. Re-programme ourselves and then the world. See our sisters, the sisterhood, as a resource; we can help them and they can help us, if we let them. If we bind together. Greet each other with love – not competition, or suspicion.

TreeSisters is a social change organisation that exists to inspire every single person to recognise their own unique role as part of the solution to global warming. It has planted over 19 million trees worldwide to help avert global warming and tackle climate change, and, fascinatingly for us women in midlife, Clare was called to the task by her own midlife awakening. She mobilised thousands of people and raised millions to plant trees.

But after a few years, she burnt out and like many founders went through a bruising process of being ejected from the organisation she created and nurtured. 'Menopause hit me like a train. I'd known I needed to slow down for a while, I had been ill and lacking energy. Then I just had to stop, go to bed. Do nothing. My own sense of mission and drive wouldn't let me stop, so my body just took over and did it for me. I stopped. I couldn't get up. I was exhausted in every possible way. I stepped away from TreeSisters, which had been my life. I am currently recovering, being still, hanging out with my amazing husband, Mark.' At the festival, when she was mobbed at the end of the session, she said, 'I'm not anyone anymore. I'm no longer a public figure. I don't represent any organisation. I don't have a website. I am just me. Putty. In the process of becoming whatever is next.'

What I admired most about that sentence was her total calm and certainty, the way she wasn't trying to give herself new titles, or new purpose or jump into the next thing. (Yes, m'lud, I was guilty on *all* those counts, when it happened to me.) Clare was just determined to be here now, as putty, in her new state of becoming whatever she was going to be next. I loved her acceptance that she was in the 'in-between', the pupa stage. Hanging on the hook, like Inanna. Whenever anyone mentioned Donald Trump or politics, or not saving the world in time, rather than getting bogged down and depressed, Clare imagined herself as a piece of kelp, or seaweed, the kind that just flows back and forwards in the current as the water flows over it. We stood up and did it together. Arms above our heads, our bodies flowing from side to side. It felt peaceful, grounding. Like the problems of the world just fell away. Go on, try it! Currently she feels a similar need 'to kelp' when there is any discussion about her future; she's happy to sit in the putty stage. I find that notion of just sitting where we are, not hurrying on to the next phase but waiting for it to find us, very refreshing and evolved. I gave her a hug and we kelped some more together, swaying in the wind, looking out over the deer park. Sharing a hug. Sisters supporting each other. Wow, it felt good.

Secret: Sometimes other women in the workplace can be our worst foes – particularly the cohort of women who were the first to climb high, because they did so by defining themselves as not like most women, as exceptional Queen bees. At a time when there was often only space for one woman at the table, we were forced to compete. But those days are over, and if we are to rise as women, we need to support each other and rise together. Next time you feel competitive about another woman, look at her with love, as your sister. If we unite against the external aggressor – at work and in the wider world – if we join together, then we are invincible.

PART FIVE

OUR BODIES

At around noon every day I gather up my swimming things – neoprene gloves, old black cossie, woolly hat, towel, Dryrobe – and drive up to the Ladies' Pond on Hampstead Heath. I have loved the water all my life, but this commitment to a daily swimming practice, in the cold water whatever the weather, all the year round, is part of my own midlife journey. A personal, daily commitment to my own well-being. To slowing down. To being in my body – and in nature.

It began during lockdown when the pond was truly a lifesaver. And I got so addicted to the endorphins, the rush of adrenaline and dopamine that flushes through me while I am doing it and afterwards, that it is now a huge part of my life and my new identity.

At the pond I notice not just the trees and birds – I've written about my feathery friends elsewhere in this book – but, always, the beauty of older female bodies. The faces may be wrinkly, the forms hidden as they trot down the muddy path to the pond under bulky jumpers or tent-like puffer coats or those ubiquitous black Dryrobes. But as they strip off, and they do, rather, *we* do, all of us standing butt-naked by the benches in the open air under the trees, whatever the weather, I can't help but notice the luminosity of the skin. The high, pert roundness of breasts under lined faces. The toned muscle in legs and arms. The fierce brightness of eyes and the charm of a wide smile in a lived-in face.

There is so much gorgeousness here in these ageing female bodies, we've just been trained by the male lens of our culture not to see it.

Do a little experiment. Next time you are watching TV or reading a magazine or looking at representations of women when out and about, count the number of women over fifty you see (who aren't Helen Mirren, Miriam Margolyes or Judi Dench). Where in real life are the billboards showing the kinds of bodies I see at the pond? Where are the magazine front covers proclaiming the beauty of real women in midlife and beyond? They are not there. Believe me. I once shot a globally famous actress for the cover of the magazine I edited. She was in her seventies, an icon; the pictures were breath-taking. When I took them to my (male) editor he said: 'God, no! Can't we have her when she was young and hot? I had her on my bedroom wall. I don't want to see her like this!' (That's what I mean by the male lens; they only want to see women they might want to fuck.)

It's not just newspapers. Where are the advertising campaigns extolling the strength and stamina of older women? The wisdom in their wrinkles or bulges? They just don't exist, even though, as I've said before, we wield significant spending power. While I was writing this book four iconic 1990s supermodels – Christy, Linda, Naomi and Cindy – appeared on the cover of *Vogue*. I hadn't even finished posting on my socials about how refreshing it was when the gendered-ageist backlash set in about them looking like 'Real Housewives going to a funeral, or a post-divorce party'.

We discussed this at a Noon women's circle. How women have been taught to judge and measure ourselves and each other. 'That is my edge,' admitted one woman. 'Where I have to consciously train my mind not to judge, to look for the beauty, to celebrate the age and wisdom in older women. We can all do that with some effort, with some conditioning. Teach ourselves not to judge other women through male eyes.'

I suppose that is what I have been doing at the pond. Cultivating a different kind of awareness. Seeking out new forms of beauty by not seeing critically. By not judging the women through my own internal-ised male lens which our culture imposes upon us every time we pick up a newspaper or magazine, turn on the TV or look at our phones.

One of the hardest things to quash is the negativity that comes from our own conditioning, how we've been taught to judge our own signs of age or 'imperfection' and those of other women with an often cruel and ruthless eye. We all do it. Often we are taught to do it by our mothers. That generation are forever criticising other women's bodies, pointing out their imperfections, starving themselves to meet an inner standard they could never measure up to. My mother is eighty now and she's still worried about being too fat (she isn't!). That generation all do it. They were brought up on the maxim 'you can never be too rich or too thin'.

Think about it. 'Have you lost weight?' is that generation's highest compliment. Appearance is always mentioned, discussed, as if that is what is most crucial to a female identity. How thin and beautiful a woman is. How she measures up to society's ideals; what mate she can attract. Many of that generation see themselves almost entirely through a male lens; it's what is called internalised misogyny. The way women are taught to judge and scrutinise other women to keep each other down, to compete for male attention, because that was where power lay/lies.

But it doesn't have to be like that. My daughters don't do this. In their generation it is rude to comment on someone else's body. Many of them have had 'issues' around eating – anorexia, bulimia, eating disorders – they know that a throwaway comment about a person's thinness or not can trigger an avalanche of inner turmoil. They don't ever comment on weight or bodies. I think, increasingly, they don't judge or measure themselves in that way. I've learnt to do the same. It is curiously liberating. Just try it – try *never* commenting on other women's bodies, or weight. It feels strange to begin with, but then it works. You just train yourself out of thinking about it, giving it centre stage. What a relief!

We can all be guilty of judging others and ourselves, of staring in the mirror with self-hatred, smoothing away our wrinkles, breathing in to remove that extra tyre. I know I do this. What would happen, I wonder, if rather than judging ourselves so harshly we tried to be loving or generous to ourselves instead? If we saw ourselves through a Queenager lens of celebration of our years and our wisdom rather than only valuing ourselves as women for our fanciability and fecundity, or hotness and fertility, as the patriarchy has taught us? After all, if we don't truly see and love ourselves and other women of our age, how can anyone else? All change starts inside each of us and spreads out in a positive vibration around the world.

I remember going for a massage when I was in my thirties, after I'd had my second kid. I was brutally out of shape, exhausted; I was living almost entirely in my head. The masseuse said to me: 'One day you'll learn to live in your body too. You'll learn to love it.' At the time I dismissed it. Twenty years later I know what she meant.

For me this midlife immersion in the physical, which started with those daily visits to the pond, is not just about fitness or machines or even healthspan. It is about a deeper embrace of the sensual. The joy of feeling sun on our face, or taking a deep breath in a beechwood, the sense of hands buried deep in compost or earth as we plant bulbs or seeds, the rhythm in our bodies of walking all day or cycling hard, the touch of fur or a pet's rough tongue on our skin, connection with another human being. As the years pass, it seems we become more grateful for the simple act of being; in this body, at this time – still here.

Beauty's impossible standards

It was a tweet that got to me. 'New Term, New Trim!' Susanna Reid, the midlife television presenter of Britain's biggest morning show, was showing off her new bob. 'At 52, I've had the CHOP. But Cher told me this morning, women should keep their hair LONG as they grow older. What do YOU think?' she asked, all chumminess.

Well, frankly, I'm fed up to the back teeth with being told what I should and shouldn't wear and what to do with my hair! I'm also tired of the only older women appearing in the mainstream being the kind who look decades younger than they really are. It semaphores that they are the only ones allowed to be seen, that the rest of us should strive – and most importantly spend – to be eternally youthful like them.

This is the male lens in action. Women seeing themselves through men's eyes. Believing that they are only valuable for their looks, for how fecund and fanciable they can make themselves. That as they age, they must sweat harder, go under the knife, try ever more desperately to cling onto youth, onto the currency of hotness. To seek and hold the male gaze. That that currency is all that matters.

This bilge is pumped out by glossy magazines, pimped by female celebrities (usually being paid by beauty brands). Now there is no end point when we are permitted to give up the beauty arms race, retire gracefully. In fact, the push to remain perpetually youthful is with us now more than ever. Surgery, tweakments, filters – an entire industry exists to encourage us to hang onto our juiciness. Anti-ageism is presented as Martha Stewart posing in a bikini on the cover of *Sports Illustrated*, at eighty – airbrushed to oblivion, wrinkles erased, looking all – fake – hot blondeness. Yet another impossible beauty standard. Surely, by the time we reach our ninth decade it should stop?

Well, yes, I'm calling 'time'. I've had at least forty years' worth of bossy style 'tips' (more like 'commands') directed my way. And I'm done. In one weekend I was bombarded with an almost endless list of 'essentials' to make my Queenager body and face acceptable. The injunctions included an article telling me exactly what kind of shapewear I should be sporting at all times (no thanks, it constricts the tummy, is hot and sweaty, and what's wrong with the odd bulge, I've had two kids and like pasta?). Whether or not I'm allowed to wear a bikini in midlife (frankly, I'll be the judge of that; if I don't want white tan lines, I'll wear a two-piece and take my top off if I feel like it). I'm told I *should* wear navy not black (kinder to the complexion), not show my bingo wings (sorry, they are my arms), or knees (ditto), and that scarves are *de rigueur* to cover wrinkly necks (who are they offending?). Oh, and apparently I *should* embrace neon bright colours and metallics as my new basics, to stay 'with it'. The rules are confusing and contradictory – perhaps that's the point.

And when it comes to our hair, it's never-ending. Apparently BTB (below the boobs) is a prerequisite for Queenagers because Gwyneth has it, and so does Sarah Jessica Parker, Beyoncé, Amal Clooney and all the nineties supermodels. Oh, and of course Cher, who says long hair is anti-ageing. One month it's 'midlife hair must be long', the next that long is witchy and it must be short. Then that we should cover up the grey, but not go too dark as lighter is good for the skin. And don't get me started on hot-pink menopausal product marketing for conditioners that prevent 'Hagrid hair'.

The truth is, this is all a load of tosh. Being a Queenager is all about freeing ourselves from everything we were told we were supposed to do, be and particularly look like. Top of the list is ditching the obligation to be 'pleasing' both physically and temperamentally. I don't know about you but I wasted far too much time providing social oil and tripping around in heels to please my older male bosses. The great thing about midlife is that we can do exactly what pleases us; my definition of Queenager is that it's whatever you want it to be. That goes for clothes and body parts too.

That freedom to be who we want to be is the essence of Queenager-hood. In our survey 60 per cent of the women agreed that: 'Now is my time, I've spent the last decades looking after everyone else, now it is time for me.' That means not doing what others want or expect but what we feel like. We also understand that, by fifty, defining ourselves by what we look like is a total waste of time. It's sweating a diminishing asset. I remember being at a grand charity ball, held in an ornate ballroom in Claridge's in central London, and looking around me at all these wealthy ladies of a certain age. They were plucked, and tweaked, and Pilates-ed up to the max, but I remember thinking what a colossal collective waste of time and energy that was. No surgeon or product – however expensive – would make them young again. They just looked like weird, distorted versions of themselves. Skin over-shiny, faces that didn't move, identikit brows. Trapped in delusion.

Of course, stay healthy and active and look and feel like you want to be – I'm a great believer in you do you. But remember, one of the great liberations of turning fifty is that by this point in our lives, however beautiful we've been, our looks are no longer the key to anything. By midlife it's time to embrace all that we are – creative, intelligent, kind, competent, experienced, loving, loved, dextrous, fit – not just the externals. It's time, Queenagers, to transcend the constant focus on our female appearance. To put it behind us. To revel in and be all that we are – freed from the pressure to be pleasing to the male eye.

I've felt that shift myself. Before lockdown I used to wear heels; I am quite short and roundish so I thought they made me look taller and more elegant. Now? No way. They hurt and if I put on a pair I can't stomp to the Tube, or walk between meetings. I suppose I could carry heels in my handbag, but you know what? I'm often heaving around my laptop and I just can't be bothered to carry stilettos or truss myself up in Spanx anymore. The days when people were looking at my body are gone. If they are meeting me now, it's for my brain and the content of my character. It's nice to look cheerful. Colourful maybe. Like a good version of ourselves. Or, as an old mentor of mine, at eighty, puts it: 'Neat and tidy – that's the best I can do.' That is fine.

It's a different way of being in the world. I'm not trying to be fanciable; I'm no longer trading on erotic capital. My aim is to be memorable, chic, comfortable and entirely myself. I love my gold Air Force trainers and my outsized gold sunglasses. I have crazy curly hair and I love a bright-green sweater. A green leather coat. Shiny green chrome nails. It's about Queenager cool, feeling confident and vibrant as you, not va-va-voom. It's a huge relief.

The truth is that confidence is what is attractive in a woman, especially as she ages. Confidence and energy. The reason we think we need to look a certain way, buy all those products, worry about our wrinkles, erase those bulges, is largely because a multibillion-dollar cosmetics industry spends inordinate sums telling us that we do. Did you know that the profit margin on beauty products is over 80 per cent? It's a licence to print money. Kirsten Miller, US author of *The Change*, a brilliant thriller about menopause, pulled the lid off this for me at a Noon Book Club session. Before she became an author, she'd worked in advertising in New York for twenty-five years.

'The truth is that billions of dollars are spent telling us we need this shampoo, or long blonde hair, or this slimming product so we look a certain way, but that's because these huge global companies want to sell you products. The truth is that it is a woman's energy, her confidence, her innate sense of herself that makes her attractive, but advertisers can't sell you that so they sell you make-up and perfume and hair products instead. But remember, that's just lies!'

I love that. Just remember: it's your hair, your face, your body – so do what feels right for you. And the rules? Sod 'em.

Tabitha James Kraan is an elegant, 55-year-old Queenager with long silver hair. She is a hairdresser in Gloucestershire, and all day, every day, she talks to midlife women about how they feel about themselves, how they would like to look. If anyone understands their programming and insecurities, it is her.

Fascinatingly, she sees real variation across the age groups, with core Queenagers, women in their fifties, being the pivot generation. 'I find that women aged sixty-five-plus who were very much brought up to value themselves on their looks are generally obsessed with looking as young as possible; these are the cohort who, if they have the cash, are straight down to the clinic to get surgery or Botox. Women in their fifties, however, are beginning to shift – they are more keen on growing old with individuality. They are often concerned about young women, often their daughters' generation, who are growing up in a world of Instagram filters … I find there is a growing sense among older women that we need to be role models for younger generations, show them how to value themselves as they age; that we need to resist the current celebrity route of Botox and surgery and dyeing our hair into oblivion and model something more self-accepting and authentic.'

I was so interested to hear Tabitha say that because it is very much what I see around me. I was out for drinks with about fifteen of my oldest friends from university. It was striking that none of the women had that Botox wind-tunnel look; we were all wearing our wrinkles with pride.

Tabitha's aim is to get her midlife clients to honour where they are. See their wrinkles as evidence of the life they have lived, the joys and sorrows they have shared. 'I want to give them confidence in who they are, what their individual strengths and qualities are, both in terms of their hair but also more broadly.' Like me at the pond, Tabitha is looking for what she calls 'the specific beauty which shows up in that woman, the detail which is their strength. We all have one! It's to get them away from the idea that "I am the sum of my looks and that is all I am" – to shift them instead into presenting as their full self, all that they are, the best version of themselves. Of course, we all want to look good but not to the point where it controls, defines or limits us, or is painful, or impeding our other choices. Those are signs that our looks are controlling us, that the surface has become too important, that we have gone too far.' This is all about unpicking the trope that little girls learn very young, that their appearance is the most important thing about them. We need to stop saying 'aren't you pretty, aren't you good' to girls and young women and praise them for being forceful, or creative, or kind, or fun. It's so easy to slip into those blue/pink stereotypes, we all do it. But the only way we change that programming is by modelling something else. I've been trying it with all my little nieces – praising them for being brave when body-surfing waves, or for their wonderful drawings, or being kind to each other. Try it.

Secret: Embrace being authentically you. It's fine to want to look nice but if it hurts, takes up huge amounts of time, money and energy and is beginning to control and dominate your life, then it's time for a change. Embrace who and what you are – wear your favourite colour, invest in some funky trainers or a bright coat. Forget the sexual arms race.

Let's just age gracefully

What is gendered ageism? For me it is where sexism and ageism collide in a double whammy. We were treated to a rant about it by no less a person than Queen Madge, the Madonna herself, after the world recoiled at her face at the 2023 Grammys.

'Once again I am caught in the glare of the ageism and misogyny that permeates the world we live in,' said Madonna in a statement posted to Instagram. 'A world that refuses to celebrate women past the age of forty-five and feels the need to punish her if she continues to be strong-willed, hard-working and adventurous.'

I felt rather wary of straying into this territory; my default is always to support other women. But with Madonna I feel strongly there is a disconnect. Isn't Madonna, by baby-fying her face, playing into the tropes of an ageist-misogynist culture? After all, the Rolling Stones don't plump their cheeks to look younger; they strut out on stage looking like wrinkly reptiles, glorying in the centuries they have clocked up between them. Surely, if Madonna really wanted to own her age, to combat ageism, to be proud about being sixty-four, she'd sing her record-breaking songs looking proudly and provocatively herself at sixty-four? She has always been a beautiful woman, why can't she look like a beautiful older woman?

I am a huge Madonna fan. I love many of her songs – she's provided the soundtrack to so much of our Queenager lives, and her cheerful, go-girl philosophy has endeared her to billions and multi-generations of women (in my family my teens and I will cheerfully sing along to Queen Madge; she is one of our in-car go-tos). Which is why I find it so sad that even Madonna can't, or won't, let herself age; won't let herself be her true sixty-something self. What kind of message does that send out to all her fans, young and old, about self-acceptance, or how to age, or that it's okay for a famous woman to have wrinkles? I find it enraging that so many women in and out of the public eye mutilate themselves in an ever more futile bid to look younger, even though it is expensive, painful and not very effective. They just end up looking weird. Talk about the law of diminishing returns. I was desperate for Madonna to buck this trend.

When it comes to this kind of facial surgery I think we all need to learn the lesson of Joan Rivers, the veteran comedienne who had over 700 cosmetic procedures on her face and body. Joan's daughter wrote after she died that her mother had 'always loathed the way she looked and suffered a constant sense of lack'. Obviously not something all that surgery could fix or she wouldn't have had so much of it. Or take Monica from *Friends*, the actress Courteney Cox, who bravely admitted she'd overdone the Botox, fillers, etc., and said she was done with it all. 'There was a time when you go: "Oh, I'm changing. I'm looking older." And I tried to chase that youthfulness for years. And I didn't realise that, oh shit, I'm looking really strange with injections and doing stuff to my face that I would never do now.' She is now sixty and says, 'There's nothing wrong with being sixty. Time goes so fast. There's no question that I am more grounded; I've learnt so much in life, what to enjoy, what to try to do more of, and what to let go of.'

Letting go of youth, embracing our Queenager-hood – that's what I'd like to see in our global female icons. An encouraging sign that we are winning the fight on valuing women for *all* that they are, not just their sexy bodies and faces, would be for older women to stop putting noxious toxins and alien agents into their faces. Men don't as a rule. Why should we? As one Queenager wrote on the Noon Instagram:

'I'm sorry that women in any walk of life feel they need to distort their faces and bodies because of sexism, ageism, racism, the patriarchy.' Hear, hear!

We need a fundamental shift here; my thinking about it goes something like this: let's consider women as being like rainbows. Our physical self is one colour. Our capacity to reproduce another. Our mind and thoughts another. Our purpose another. Our capacity to care and love, another. Our creativity, our kick-ass will, our energy, our striving, our spirituality, all more amazing colours. But too often our culture ignores the full spectrum of all that we are, seeing only the man-pleasing surface or the womb. Wow, that sounds very *Handmaid's Tale*, I know, but Margaret Atwood said when she wrote that book that everything in it had happened in some society at some point in history. Similarly, everything I am trying to do with this book is to challenge that lens, unpick it. To understand that every time we cause ourselves pain trying to chase the elixir of youth to serve the male lens, we do ourselves and our sex a disservice. We are failing to see the whole rainbow of who and what we are and how much all those other things matter.

We play the patriarchy's game when we value ourselves on our looks, our youthfulness. It's not surprising we do this. We've been taught since we were old enough to learn to value the bits that are covetable to men. Little girls are constantly praised for being 'pretty' or 'good'. We are taught to internalise misogyny, to hate and judge ourselves for getting older. To look in the mirror and loathe our wrinkles, worry about how we measure up to other women, judge other women, put each other down.

Everywhere women turn, we're exhorted to see ourselves through a male lens; to hate our cellulite, worry about not having a beach-ready body or whatever stupid characteristic some women's magazine or self-hating female columnist has chosen to make up that week – see cankles, or bingo wings, or worrying about wrinkles, or does my bum look big in this. Believe me on this – I had a front-row seat in the media as this was all going on.

The terrifying thing about fear of ageing is how young it starts. A 51-year-old told me how she'd taken her 21-year-old daughter for Botox. A 25-year-old told me she was worried about her wrinkles. A Queenager said her 18-year-old was having her lips plumped and injected into a trout pout. Instagram filters have a lot to answer for; Gen Z is more terrified of ageing than ever because they live their lives online, constantly posting images of themselves. Their fear of not looking perfect is crucifying.

This is insane and dangerous nonsense. It infuriates me. The whole point of feminism was for women not to be defined by their biology; how, in 2024, can so many twenty-somethings be having their lips blown up with fillers or having toxins injected into their lovely young faces to block non-existent lines? The problem with misogyny is it doesn't go away, it mutates. The current pornified culture makes nearly all young people feel inadequate in their most intimate lives. At least for us it was only paper magazines and the telly; now it's constant social media scrutiny (and full faces of make-up at all times as a result) and a generation taught about sex by online pornography and its norms. Enforcing even more impossible and pervasive beauty standards.

We need to deprogramme ourselves, to stop seeing ourselves through an ageist, misogynistic lens. I know that Madonna is an artist and claims that she is making 'artistic' choices about how she presents herself. But still, I wish she would reconsider. Let's just grow old. There is so much beauty in that.

No one exemplifies this more than my friend Rachel Peru. I love her story because it is so positive, such a beacon of a shift we can all make if we so choose. Rachel became a curve and lingerie model at fifty. She is no size zero and for much of her life was unhappy with her body and her figure.

She left school without any career plans and worked in retail for a decade, paying the bills. By thirty, she felt unfulfilled despite being married with two kids and another on the way. 'I kept thinking: Is this it? Is this going to be the sum of my life.' At thirty-nine, '[something] changed inside, a new sense of urgency within me that I couldn't ignore'. Rachel divorced the husband she had been with since she was sixteen. 'To say that the following few years were a rollercoaster of emotions is an understatement. Total grief for the life I'd left behind was mixed with pure excitement to find out who I really was – and what that person might be capable of being and doing.'

She chose a word for her next decade: brave.

She started her own vintage clothing business, selling at fairs every weekend and creating a website. This led to her modelling at a local Macmillan Cancer Support fashion show in her native Yorkshire. 'Standing behind the stage waiting to walk down the catwalk was nerve-racking. A negative loop was running in my head: What if I fall in my heels? What will people think I look like? What if I make a fool of myself?' But the reality was exhilarating and liberating.

'As soon as it was over I just wanted to do it again. I walked down that runway feeling like I owned it. I felt proud of my curvy body and grey hair and realised that I was good enough, just as I was in that moment. I'd spent years struggling to like my body; it stopped me from joining in with so many things, from trying new sports to always dreading clothes shopping. There's a distinct lack of me in any photographs from when my children were younger ... I never thought about modelling professionally. It just wasn't on my radar. After all, I was a curvy size 14/16, five-foot-seven, 44-year-old woman with grey hair – not your stereotypical model material.'

Rachel decided to try making modelling a career and sent some basic images off to model agencies. She got signed quickly by a London agency. 'My imposter syndrome was very real and there have been lots of times when I could have given up. But I'm glad to say that that word – *brave* – carried me forward. Within the first year, I modelled swimwear alongside the iconic curve model Ashley Graham and American singer Lizzo. I've finally found my passion and purpose. My favourite bookings are swimwear and lingerie campaigns because the feedback I receive from other women over forty, who still don't feel visible or represented in advertising, is always such a boost to any lack of confidence I may have. Yes, change and personal growth can be hard, scary and messy, and it's a rollercoaster, but it is also exhilarating.'

Rachel now models all over the world and loves the way what she is doing inspires other women of her age. 'I'm fifty-two now and this decade's word is "ambition".' It sounds like the title of a Madonna song – maybe Madge should try it.

Gendered ageism needs to be tackled and driven out of our own unconscious and from society. We do that by telling new stories, pointing out that the current story is misogynist and ageist; that it needs a new script. That is what I am trying to do in this book. We need to tackle our own inner ageism, to stop ourselves looking at and judging and hating our wrinkles; to instead view our bodies with love that they continue to serve us, that they have carried us this far. That we are lucky to be here.

Secret: Emancipate yourself from the male lens which makes us judge ourselves and value ourselves by men's metrics of hotness and fertility. Women are rainbows – celebrate all that you are.

This beautiful body of mine

For aeons women's bodies have been used as ornaments, as eye candy for men. 'Brighten up the page, love!' as the old editor used to shout – meaning, put in a picture of a pretty girl. Just think about how cars were sold for ages, with naked young women draped over their bonnets. The girl promised as an extra treat, like a fruit basket which comes with the car.

We cannot fail to be affected by this, particularly as our bodies age and draw further and further away from the 'ideal' our society pushes on us. In fact, I've always felt there was a freedom in being nothing like that ideal. The women I've known who have been most worried about perfection, and measured themselves against it constantly and harshly, have been those closest to it – tall, slim, beautiful; they become tortured by not being quite good enough, any imperfection is exaggerated. I see it now. It is my most beautiful friends, the ones whose looks were always intrinsic to their identity, who come and confess they are considering an eye lift, or a tweakment. The great beauties never seem to recognise that they were it … whatever 'it' was. 'It' didn't make them happy, though; like the closer you got to 'it', the more evanescent it was, the further away it became.

I was always miles away from 'it' – how we were supposed to look according to the prevailing fashion for beauty. I've always been buxom and curvaceous. At my thinnest a size 12/14 on the bottom but always a HH cup on top, necessitating bras that can be worn as head-dresses with very supportive straps. I've never had any complaints from men or a lack of takers. It's the internalised misogyny of the female gaze that I've felt found me lacking. Like my chubby thighs or tummy rolls were an afront to them.

I'm used to that reaction. From when I was eight, my parents felt I was too fat. I could feel my mother's eyes judging the contents of my plate; I'd clear the table and finish off the odd potato surreptitiously on the way to the dishwasher. My mum bought a book: *Cooking to Make Kids Slim*, which had a sad-looking plump girl on the front gazing disconsolately at the scales she was standing on. God, I hated that book.

I was forced to take 'healthy' lunches to school (so I couldn't eat custard). Those Tupperware boxes full of lukewarm grated carrot and cottage cheese haunt me still. Carrying them into lunch was the equivalent of wearing a scarlet letter; except this one said: too fat, problematic.

In my teens it got worse. I was sent to a diet doctor in Harley Street. I nicknamed him Dr Slimy – because he was. He had a tufty beard and always got a bit too close when he weighed me. His laugh was annoying and he said 'super-duper' a lot. He put me on amphetamine pills to limit my appetite. I took them for several years. They worked a bit like these new Wegovy injections; I wasn't hungry, I was a bit manic. I was still never thin (though when I see photographs of myself then I was a totally normal size, yet I was made to feel like a heifer).

This very focused attention from my parents on my weight was unhelpful to say the least. My dad left when I was five and one of the few times I saw him alone after that was when he took me to the fat doctor. The fact that my parents, who didn't agree on anything much, both thought my size was an issue made me feel bad about myself. Lacking. Not good enough. Too much. Like there needed to be less of me, like I needed fixing to be lovable. Even to them.

I am pretty confident now but, even so, appearance can be my Achilles' heel. Before a big keynote speech or TV interview, my anxiety goes not to what I will say (I always feel pretty confident about that) but to what I will wear. I can lie in bed working through the upsides and downsides of possible outfit combinations for literally hours, trading off comfort (flat shoes, comfy knickers) for glamour, meaning looking thinner (heels, Spanx). Appearance becomes the sticky heart of my nerves around an event. And, yes, I berate myself for this obsession with form rather than substance. I know how stupid it is. Particularly now as a 52-year-old woman when nobody is looking at me anyway. Where probably the best we can do is to be cheerful, elegant and not frighten the horses, perhaps with a flash of verve and personality to show we are still alive. But basically, as women we have been programmed to be relentlessly concerned about our appearance; just observe how often you tell small girls they are pretty, or you like their dress. I am no exception to that rule. I just want to be honest about how, even when we understand and rail against the forces that conspire against us as Queenagers, it is only human to also feel them given the world we have grown up in.

But I've learnt that the best antidote to all this body-size crap is a health scare. I went to have a mole on my face investigated by the doctor – who referred me to a specialist. Once there, they studied my body all over for more dodgy moles, deciding my cheek was fine but a black spot on my shoulder required removal. I rocked up at the clinic for the biopsy feeling blasé – and was then ambushed by how much it hurt and how weak I felt. I was forbidden from swimming for two weeks (bad). And had a worrying ten days trying not to think about what I would do if it was skin cancer. Luckily, I was okay. I cried when I got the all-clear letter.

But one of the upsides of the whole business is that I have been thinking about my body in a whole new grateful way; not for what it looks like, or if there could be less of it, but for how happy and fortunate I am that it still carries me about and is, generally, active and healthy. It can propel me up and over Moroccan mountains, swim me round coral reefs, ski downhill, take me to the beloved pond.

I've had one of those periods where I've been reminded that health really is our most precious of commodities. But it is one of the salient parts of being fifty that people around us aren't so lucky. It's like wink murder, you never know who will be hit next. I got a weird frisson of fear and premonition at dinner with a friend when she told me she had to go back to hospital for more tests on her womb. I didn't say anything, but I hugged her hard when she left and I shed a little tear in my car on the way home. Not because she is sick but because the idea of losing someone so dear to me, even the vague possibility of it, was so scary and sad. And then on a whim, feeling a little trepidatious, I called another close old colleague, who I knew was in the middle of radiotherapy and chemo for breast cancer, who started off sounding low but, after we'd exchanged a bit of scurrilous gossip and reminisced a bit, was so funny and raw and real and lovable that I came off the phone glad I'd called. It was probably one of our best-ever chats, the culmination of so much shared time and endeavour in the past. I know I cheered her up but she helped me too. I should have called her sooner.

These tough times come to us all. They are as much a part of the Queenager experience as the joy of a new tribe or finding our purpose. The prevalence of these big conversations, the part they play in our lives, are not talked about very much. But I reckon we owe it to our friends – in fact, it is probably the key part, the definition, of being a friend at this point – not to shirk the difficult conversations or avoid them (tempting) but to lean in and use our love, affection and intimate knowledge of them to help them cope. Often just being there, checking in, helps. Not necessarily talking about 'it' all the time, but allowing that to come up if necessary. And maybe sending a little treat through the post: brownies, or flowers, or a book, or even vegan cookies. There's nothing like a little surprise, a thoughtful gesture … even a note, a text message or a meaningful emoji. It can mean so much.

But most important – I think – is being prepared to go there, to really talk. To have the sort of conversations where you kind of have to pinch yourself that it is really happening, where you are talking to a friend about something big and real and scary and you need to be there for them, to hold space for them in that moment, let them express their fears, help them feel safe and heard.

I think we Queenagers are good at that; we've all been through enough to know that sometimes that kind of engagement is necessary. That it is just life. Maybe being a real grown-up is doing that. Comforting those in pain, supporting them through the difficult stuff. Indeed, often in the weeds of those conversations – the type where we just really try to be there for the other person, with love – are some of the sweetest times we ever have as humans. That point of light, of connection, of love in the darkness, really is the brightest we ever burn. These are some of the loveliest soul-to-soul exchanges we ever have. True, honest, loving – reaching out across fear to bring comfort, to let them know we are there and we love them, that they matter. Let's all try to be rather un-British and embrace these chats rather than shying away.

Secret: If there is a conversation you need to have, or someone you can comfort – do it!

The big C

It was meant to be a fun night out. We were meeting for what the kids call 'pres' – pre-event drinks – at my house before going out to dance to the Stereo MCs at a club in Kings Cross. Friends were coming from out of town; we'd been looking forward to it. But when Liza arrived I could see something was wrong. She has bright-green eyes, usually they flash with fun. Tonight the lights were out. She seemed fragile, older, sad. I took her upstairs to the spare bedroom and gave her a hug. 'You all right?' She started to cry. That day had been spent inside an MRI scanner and having umpteen painful mammograms. The news was bad: she had breast cancer, she was going to need surgery, three months of chemo and radiotherapy. Her husband looked like he'd been punched. I hugged them both, made a bad joke about the chug, chug, CHUUUUGGG of the scanner, which made them laugh. We talked about how brilliant the treatments are these days, how the doctors said that she would be okay.

I tried to be cheerful but this was close, too close. Especially because only a few days before I'd been on the phone for an hour with another friend whose hair was falling out from chemo, who had forgotten her scarf and 'terrified the old dears in the village shop' with her baldness. She was being so funny and brave but in the quiver of her voice I could sense her terror. She talked about those moments in our lives when we get news we don't want, where there is a time before and a time after. And a chasm yawns between the two; unbridgeable. There is no going back. It reminds me of that quote from *The Bridge of San Luis Rey* by Thornton Wilder: 'There is a land of the living and a land of the dead and the bridge is love, the only survival, the only meaning.'

But there is survival. And hope. Which is why Lindsey's story of coming through breast cancer is so inspirational.

As we spoke over Zoom, Lindsey told me that it was between Christmas and New Year, while she was shaving her armpits, that she found a lump under her arm. 'I was forty-five. I rang the doctor and went for a mammogram two weeks later. They did a biopsy quickly. But in between seeing the GP and the consultant I found another lump in my breast. It was funny. I was lying in bed with my husband, fooling around, saying to him how hard it was to find lumps in the breast, demonstrating comically how you were supposed to do it: you know, squishing the breasts between your hands. And then I found one. Not so funny.'

She had another mammogram and this time it wasn't just the consultant who saw her but a whole team. 'It's not good,' they said. 'Grade 2, stage 2. We need to do a lumpectomy, clear the lymph nodes.'

That was, she says, the worst moment. 'I was convinced I was going to die. It was all I could think about. I'm going to die. I went home and was clinging to my husband through the night saying, "I don't want to die, I don't want to die."' Fortunately the morning brought clarity. She decided to focus not on death, but only on the positive: the doctors had said it was treatable. 'I hung onto that like a life raft.'

She went back to hospital again. This time for a week. They'd found seventeen cancerous lymph nodes plus cancerous cells in the margins. There was another deep tumour growing right into her ribs. It was stage 3. They had to take out everything. But they still said they could treat her so she clung onto that.

Lindsey had six months of chemo and twenty-five sessions of

radiotherapy. It was intense. But what I love about her story is her attitude. 'Apart from that one night of despair I am a glass-half-full kind of gal. Thinking negatively just takes you to a bad place. I tried to enjoy myself as much as I could. Even to see the funny side of the bit of wire they put around my tiny breast to show the lump. I just thought: cut it all off! I even chuckled to myself.'

It is that kind of black humour that often gets us through tough times; like getting the giggles at a funeral, or being able to laugh with someone even as they are dying. Lindsey was very open about her illness. 'I didn't want anyone to feel weird around me or that any subjects were off limits. I spoke to my kids about it right at the beginning and said the doctors thought I would be all right. They were okay after that.'

Her worst moment – and I know this is true of other friends too – was when she lost her beautiful long hair. 'At the gym I remember putting conditioner into my hair and it all fell out, it was tangled round my fingers. I couldn't get rid of it, I couldn't find a sink. It was like Lady Macbeth – "out, damned spot, out, I say!"' After that she had it all shaved off and covered her bald head with bandanas and colourful scarves.

Often it is when we realise how lucky we are in respect to others that the truth of our situation emerges. Lindsey described removing her bandana at the gym next to a young woman, who removed her own scarf too. 'She was also bald and she told me how brave I was and then said sadly: "Your hair will grow back when you get better, mine won't because I have alopecia."'

After that, Lindsey says she 'kind of stopped caring about wearing a scarf. I just decided to be me in all my glory. People feed off your energy and my matter-of-factness helped everyone around me.'

There is a pause, and I can see Lindsey smiling all the way from New York. 'All that was nine years ago. I'm off all the medication now. It's nearly ten years. There is life after cancer!' So, what did she learn from the experience? 'That my friends really were my friends. That I loved my husband. They all came through for me. I didn't lose anyone. That made me feel very sure and certain of my life and the judgements I'd made of the people around me.' She says there was even an upside which will resonate with so many of us. 'I always had big guilt, I'd worry about things and endlessly seek approval. These days, I don't. There's not enough time for that kind of self-doubt. Now I ask for forgiveness, not permission or approval. I ask myself: what's the worst that can happen if I do this? And you know what? Compared to having stage 3 cancer, it's never that bad! So I just get on with it. My imposter syndrome has gone. I have more confidence.'

You always wonder if something like this happened whether you would be the same person – what I find truly uplifting about Lindsey's story is that she came through her illness not just the same but, as she puts it, 'Better! After the cancer, I feel I know myself and I have a lot more confidence and solidity in myself, my choices, that I am living the right life. That feels good.'

I'm glad to say that my own friend Liza has also come through her treatment and is well again. She's sporting a very natty cropped hairdo, has allowed it to go grey, and looks gamine and mischievous. Most importantly she is still here. Her birthday is just after Christmas so her husband organised a surprise party. We are a close group of friends; we go camping together every year, our kids have grown up together, like a big unruly mass of cousins. I told my kids there was a party for Liza. They both had other things to do that day but they cancelled them instantly. When she walked into her sitting room and saw us all there, she cried. So did all the rest of us; there wasn't a dry eye in the house. In that moment, seeing her well, in her purple dress next to her purple-adorned Christmas tree, we all let out a collective breath – she was alive. We all love her. We all felt how close we had come to losing her. How happy we all were that she was still among us.

Our bodies are miracles – they anchor us to the glory of being right here, right now.

Secret: The cancer brought Lindsey clarity: it made her alive to the present moment. That when it came to her one wild and precious life, she was on the right track. Could you say the same? That you are alive, on the right track, living the right life?

Menopause – more than a hot flush

It would be impossible to write about female bodies in midlife and not mention menopause. Indeed, during the last few years in the UK at least, 'the change', as it used to euphemistically be known, has gone from being taboo to ubiquitous. This is largely down to the brilliant campaigning work of an old journalist friend of mine, Kate Muir, who had – in her own words – 'a car crash' of a menopause and wrote a book, *Everything You Need to Know About the Menopause (but were too afraid to ask)*, and produced a documentary. The latter was fronted by TV presenter Davina McCall, who also wrote a bestselling book, *Menopausing*, and in the aftermath of the books and documentary, Kate and Davina created such a huge national conversation that there was a 35 per cent uptick in prescriptions for HRT – hormone replacement therapy – in the UK. Which proves to me that storytelling really can change the world!

In fact, Britain leads the way in this conversation thanks to the efforts of campaigning Queenager MPs such as Carolyn Harris, Parliament's menopause champion, who has been on this since 2018 and now pushes for the conversation to be more inclusive. 'I was talking to a group of shop workers about menopause,' she told me, 'and one of them said: "Aren't you posh having a menopause!" Those are the ones that I really worry about, the women working all day on low incomes, without access to treatment or information. They end up not on HRT but antidepressants, really suffering.' She is right. The poorest parts of the UK have half the number of women being prescribed HRT as the richest ones. There is also a massive discrepancy in the treatment received by BAME women, who tend to have earlier menopause and worse symptoms and are less diagnosed (there is also a dearth of research into this). As Dr Nighat Arif, our Noon doctor, explains: 'In my community – of Pakistani origin – there is no word for menopause, it is just "barren".' That is unfortunately still the case in too many parts of the world. All women will go through menopause, yet in the UK until 2023 it was not mandatory for doctors to have menopause training.

I believe that the rise of the menopause conversation – the fact that here in the UK many businesses have menopause champions and the media is awash with actresses and TV presenters telling us all about their hot flushes – is the first roar of the Queenagers, our new demographic of empowered midlife women. But it is important to keep the conversation going and not let it fade, because the real-life suffering of women who have what Kate dubbed 'a car-crash menopause' is all too real. And there is still huge ignorance about the topic. Dr Nighat says that 25 per cent of women have really troublesome menopausal symptoms (serious depression, sleeplessness, heart palpitations) and too many still don't get access to the treatment they need. This is Kate Muir's account. It still packs a mega punch.

Kate says that until she met the menopause and its dastardly precursor, the perimenopause, she thought she was capable of coping with anything. But, she says, 'My passage through midlife's magnificent shit show has been an education which both put me in my place, and helped me understand how tough that place is for others.' The more she finds out about what happens to women in menopause – physically, mentally, medically and culturally – the more she is on a war footing. 'My extensive campaigning around all of this stems from my own menopause experience – less a journey and more a full *Thelma & Louise* car crash.'

Kate's story began with heart palpitations and erratic heartbeats in the middle of the night. 'There was a sudden, fast, panicky pounding in my chest and a tightness in my throat. I still had my periods, but I also had a few hot flushes.' But – and this will be familiar to many women – her GP decided she was too young to be menopausal and sent her for an electrocardiogram instead. 'I'm a runner,' says Kate. 'My heart was fine. The doctor's diagnosis was "too much coffee". Of course, now that I've read umpteen menopause manuals, I know that those harmless palpitations were a classic sign of falling oestrogen levels, and are reported by 11 per cent of women. My doctor, however, did not. That's because menopause – and perimenopause – was not then a compulsory module in GPs' training.'

Kate was furious that no one had ever told her that perimenopause, the years when oestrogen levels begin to dip before our periods cease completely, was a thing. 'But it's the elephant in the powder room. I somehow thought perimenopause was a relatively symptomless pre-menopause. But there are oestrogen receptors in every part of your body, and if fluctuating hormones are sending erratic electrical signals to your heart and internal thermostat, what peculiar messages might they be sending to your mind?'

Soon Kate found herself in the midst of a classic midlife clusterfuck. She was raising three children, had a full-time job (as a film critic at my old newspaper, *The Times*; I was her editor for a happy year or so) and, on top of all that, she'd been going up and down to her native Scotland to help take care of her ailing mum. The pressure got too great.

'I walked out of what seemed to be a stable marriage. It felt selfish, shameful and unstoppable. I also unexpectedly changed jobs, risking my career. I just couldn't cope.' As the psychotherapist and writer Suzie Orbach puts it: 'The menopause arrives, seeking out our vulnerabilities like a guided missile, just as we need all our strength to cope with daily life.'

Kate describes perimenopause as 'feeling puppeted by forces beyond your control. Hormones play good cop, bad cop: soothing you one minute, abandoning you the next, depriving you of sleep, breaking you down. It can really mess with your mental health. When the nurturing hormones oestrogen and progesterone start disappearing, that often leaves testosterone powerfully dominant, until that goes too.'

Another *Times* writer, the columnist Caitlin Moran, wrote about the fading of oestrogen in perimenopause as the end of 'having "lady forgiveness" left in your tank. Instead there is growing anger. You want to meet up with your coven of similarly menopausal friends, all of you stoking each other's fires of outrage.'

Our Noon research shows what many of us instinctively feel – that as we hit midlife, after several decades of putting everyone else first, it is once again our time. 'The self that emerges after the caring mummy-hormones begin to disappear can be liberating as well as terrifying,' says Kate. I would say amen to that!

Some women have graceful midlife transitions – they use the jealous-making phrase 'Oh, I sailed through menopause,' and communicate brilliantly with their partners. Many recalibrate their lives, frolic with natural remedies and embrace the idea that the menopause is a 'passage to power'. In Leslie Kenton's book of that name, she suggests that during this transformation of her body and her life, a woman 'needs the knowledge of the soul – access to myths, symbols and rituals which help her reconnect with the deepest levels of intuition and instinct'.

Kate, however, says she didn't need symbols or herbal remedies but HRT. 'My hair was falling out, my memory was short-circuiting, my hot flushes were actually demonic possession, but when I asked about hormone replacement therapy I was only given synthetic progestins when my body was screaming for oestrogen.'

A menopause odyssey ensued, involving private clinics who fleeced her with unregulated drugs that eventually made her sicker, until she finally met Dr Louise Newson, a campaigning menopause specialist who got her on the right balance of hormones.

'The more I found out,' Kate says, 'the more I got incensed by the ignorance and inequality and the disregard for older women's quality of life.'

As a result of her experience, Kate, with Dr Newson, established the Menopause Charity, designed to help the 13 million menopausal women in the UK get safer information and HRT. 'Inequality is coupled with medical sexism, which fails to take account of the latest medical research, and leaves women to keep calm and carry on.'

Kate also says, 'But, in a wider way, going through menopause has taught me something new and humbling: that I couldn't always work to fix everything, I couldn't always cope, and that sometimes an outside force, like a hormonal tsunami, is unstoppable. This has certainly been a "passage to power", but it's not the passage I expected.'

Now she wants other midlife women to know the facts about menopause so their own years of change can be about metamorphosis not misery. 'I don't want other women to have to drive off the cliff like I did before picking themselves up.'

Some of the most popular talks and speeches I've given have been about unpicking what it means to be a woman in midlife. I gave a talk to a room full of advertisers at London Adweek one year about why midlife women want to be seen as Queenagers, not walking hot flushes. As the profile of menopause has been raised and it has gone from being taboo to, in some places, almost ubiquitous (among a certain brand of white female celebrities anyway, not to mention those cashing in on the hot-pink menopausal gold rush in Europe and the US), not all women are on board.

It is a difficult one to untangle because of the stigma that has raged around this conversation for so long. It is also increasingly becoming a workplace issue, with one in ten women aged fifty to sixty-four said to be leaving their jobs because of menopause.

According to Noon's Dr Nighat Arif, an expert in women's health, around a quarter of women suffer terribly with the menopause, to the extent that they can become suicidally depressed and, as well as mood swings and anxiety, suffer debilitating physical symptoms too, including heart palpitations, hot flushes, muscle aches and exhaustion. A raft of employment tribunals are proof that employers need to do more to help women survive the pinch points of the change.

For decades menopause has been discussed only in hushed whispers, generations of women have suffered in silence, ill-served by GPs who received little training in the condition (thanks to campaigning this is beginning to change). Against this background, companies acknowledging that menopause really is a thing, appointing menopause ambassadors and taking women's symptoms seriously, is just natural justice and long overdue.

But we must be careful we don't kill with kindness. By viewing Queenagers through an exclusively menopausal lens we can forget that they are also experienced and skilled workers, with huge amounts to offer. In the growing hullaballoo about symptoms such as hot flushes, sleepless nights and brain fog, we don't want to lose sight of the significant resource we older women are. In a survey carried out for Noon.org.uk with Vision Express in 2022, we found that 78 per cent of women in this bracket *don't* want to be branded as menopausal. It stands to reason: my teenage daughters would never be referred to as 'menstrual'. And we'd never say to a midlife man, 'You're in the Viagra years, welcome to the limp-dick club!'

Similarly, women in their fifties don't want to be seen purely as walking hot flushes, hysterical bundles of hormones. The whole point of feminism was for women to escape their biology; for the womb not to be their destiny. There is more to us than our physicality! It seems convenient for companies to put women into a menopausal box, a hot, sweaty, biological holding pen, just as they vie for power. It can be killing with kindness. Making us weak and exceptional, bodied, other, just when we could be taking the reins. How unsurprising that corporations have leapt on it: there is no perfect age for a woman leader. Twenties – too young; thirties – likely to have a baby; forties – ditto plus perimenopausal; fifties – hot flushes; sixties – past it. Of course this is rubbish. It is well documented that women get an energy surge post-menopause. With the kids flown (if they have them) and elderly parents often in care, women are finally free to get their heads down and pursue careers with purpose and dedication. We even have the health now to do that. But what do we get? Gendered ageism. The view of society that we are past it. Unpleasing. No longer pulchritudinous. A bit bolshy. Hard to have around. How convenient for all those men who have been running the world in their sixties and seventies forever … this needs challenging. Science has extended the runway, granted us more time. Now society needs to let us step up. We need to clear out outdated notions of women shrivelling and disappearing. The third quarter can be our Queenager prime. That is the intention of this book. To change the narrative about older women to one that sees us coming into our power, being recognised for our experience and wisdom later in life. This extends the possibilities for all women – younger women love this narrative. It deserves to be heard. This is the Queenager Revolution.

Secret: I am so grateful to campaigners like Kate Muir who have brought heretofore buried information about menopause into the light, so we can all access the help we need. But while that medical knowledge is crucial, it is not the only thing going on for women at this point. We Queenagers are more than our hormones, more than our menopause. Don't forget that. Yes, we want doctors to give us the right medication. Yes, we want employers not to fire us if we need time off for our menopausal symptoms. But equally we want to be seen for all that we are, not to be dismissed as 'hysterical' just as we finally come into our Queenager power.

It's never too late to start

The crunch of snow, the swish of skis. In front of me eight Queenagers are making their way down a mountain. Above, the north face of the Eiger sits watching, enigmatic, unflinching, unchanging. The women ski ahead, some expert, elegant in their technique, including my mother who, at eighty, is a miracle of possibility. Others have just taken up the sport. I am full of admiration for them, for strapping wooden planks onto their feet and slithering down an alien steep slope for the first time, way beyond the age of fifty.

Using our bodies like this, finding new passions in midlife, is important not just for fitness, to keep us alive, use it or lose it, but because trying something new, falling down, honing a new technique, a fresh way of being in the world, is so crucial to staying young, by which I mean staying open to life and possibility.

When we learn a new skill the brain cannot wander. Trying to master skiing, or paddle-boarding, or surfing, or tennis, or pickleball, or anything we have never done before, forces us into the now. Whizzing down mountains I find myself saying 'Wheeee!', making spontaneous, childlike exultations of joy, laughing at the sheer sensation of speed and sunshine and space. The clergymen who first skied in Switzerland said that being in the mountains made them feel closer to God. Looking out across the Jungfrau, towards the towering mountains of the Lauterbrunnen Wall, high snowy peaks stretching as far as I can possibly see, I feel almost tearful with the beauty. Giddy with the sensation.

On our last morning the two newbies who have never skied before insisted on cramming in every last minute. Our train departs at 2pm for Zurich, at 1pm we are still on the mountain. 'I just never want to stop, it is like magic, like flying ... and I am so proud of myself for learning to do it, I never want to do anything else,' says Kitty, eyes flashing with the passion of a true convert. A zealot.

Coming into our bodies, getting them to learn something new. Being in the fresh air and nature and most of all in the moment – this is what we need to do as Queenagers. It's like forming those new muscle memories; learning a new skill gives us a pathway, a map to follow to other new behaviours in our life. It's like a positive kind of addiction to all that could be to come – a sense that life is not narrowing down, but expanding. Rhonda told me how she had taken up rowing during the pandemic, that by doing so she'd dropped two stone, gained muscle she'd never had and a whole community of new friends on the River Thames. In lockdown it got her out of bed and out of her flat and her loneliness. The river, the boat, the oars, the erg offered succour on so many levels. Sport, movement, being in our bodies, show us that we can live wide and free, in novelty and joy, doing new things in our fifties and beyond. That what we learn by taking up a new sport in our bodies is also then a pathway, a reminder that we can also learn and innovate in other parts of our lives.

It is not just my Queenagers in Switzerland. Danielle lived in California and had spent decades enviously watching surfers ride the waves off the Pacific coast. But it was when her kids left home, with menopause pending, that she finally decided it was time to stop sitting on the beach watching and get into a wetsuit and join them.

It wasn't easy – the obstacles of learning to surf were daunting: the icy 10-degree water of northern California; the scary, unpredictable waves; the wobbly, narrow surfboard and, last but by no means least, what she called 'the unceasing negative, hypochondriac voice in my head'.

In those first punishing weeks of falling and getting sucked under by crashing waves, she had two rules: 'One, trust my surf instructors when they told me what to do; and, two, keep driving back out to Marin County for more lessons no matter how discouraged and beat up I felt each time.'

And, after two dozen lessons, two women's surf retreats and many hours of driving 40 miles in the dark from Berkeley over Mount Tamalpais to reach the beach at dawn, she can 'paddle mightily into rising green waves, pop onto my feet and ride a wave as it peaks and rolls, often hooting with joy, my arms upstretched in victory'.

Like many of us who find a new physical passion in midlife, Danielle has really got the bug. She now surfs religiously two to three times a week with a group of fellow Queenagers who have also recently taken it up. One of her fellow surfers is a marine researcher with deep respect for the ocean after decades of studying it; one learnt to surf in her late forties after overcoming stage 4 breast cancer; one is her best friend of thirty years, who has revived her brief teenage surf experience from Long Island; and one says the day she gives up surfing is the day she wants to stop living.

The women trade text messages all week long about wind, swell and tide forecasts, then meet at the beach parking area at first light. There they wrestle into thick wetsuits, wax their longboards and scamper across the freezing sand to the water's edge to stretch their creaky bodies while surveying the best spot on the horizon to take off into the waves.

When Danielle set out on this beginner's journey a year ago, she says she suspected surfing would bring her joy. 'But what I didn't anticipate was how quickly I would become obsessed by it. How surfing for even just an hour or two wipes my mind clean and fills me with a Zen-like body calm that lasts all day. I didn't realise how intensely I would want to surf every day – or how quickly I would turn my life around to centre it on surfing.'

She is not alone. There is a 23,000-strong Women Who Surf Facebook group alongside many Insta feeds and the Traveler Surf Club. And that spell that daily immersion in a body of water casts on those of us who do it is incredibly familiar to me. Before long it becomes essential not just to the course of a day, but to one's well-being.

'I think this sudden fall into surfing addiction is because, as my middle-aged ovaries shut down and collagen drains from my face and colour from my hair, there is something new and powerful blooming inside me – something that grows stronger each week. For the last decade I was becoming invisible as a middle-aged woman. But now I feel more beautiful and stronger than I have in decades. For sure, the fear, self-doubt and hypochondria persist. The negative, doom-expectant voice in my head remains in constant battle with my desire to improve my surf skills. Each time I surf – especially at a new beach where I've never surfed before – I experience this rollercoaster of emotions: "I can't do this. How can I even call myself a surfer? Why do I tell everyone I can surf? I should just quit now." And then – after taking deep breaths and placing my palms on the surface of the water to pause and reset – I catch my first wave of the day. As I paddle back out to the line-up after that first ride, I weep tears of joy and say aloud to myself: "I can surf! Mommy can surf!"'

So what lesson does Danielle have for other women in their fifties facing a pivot, or not quite sure what to do next? 'Surfing has not only helped me grow my physical skills but my capacity for bravery,' she says. 'One thing I know for certain is how grateful I am that I turned my long-held dream of surfing into a reality. It's worth looking inside yourself to find your own long-held dreams; choose one and act on it. Start today – your time is now.'

Secret: You are never too old and it is never too late to learn something new. Trying a physical challenge in midlife is a great way to rewire neural pathways and boost confidence more broadly. If my mum can still ski at 80, you can do something you haven't tried before too.

Sex gets better with age

I am lying in a yurt. Outside the sun is shining. In here it is hot and it smells of sweat and roses. Around me women aged from twenty to seventy are lying on rugs and cushions. There is a tautness in the air, a tension. The workshop is entitled 'Sacred Self-Pleasure' – designed to deprogramme us from guilt, shame or the urge for our sexuality to be performative. We go round a circle and woman after woman reveals the trauma that separates them from enjoying, or feeling comfortable in their bodies. Many women talk about how they had been told not to touch themselves because it was 'dirty'. When they do masturbate many feel shame – or approach it as a quick release to be got through as fast as possible and forgotten. Not all. A few talk about delightful-sounding self-care rituals involving candles and slowly, slowly bringing themselves to arousal. But most said they hadn't the time, energy or capacity to indulge themselves like that. They had four kids, or jobs – or elderly parents, or all of the above. Many of the Queenagers hadn't realised that that kind of indulgent self-pleasure was even a thing they *could* do.

Madalaine, the sexologist running the workshop, asks us to think about what our bodies like during sex, what they want, what pleasure is for each of us. Many of the women say they don't know what they want or like. Sex for them has always been about what their – usually – male partners want, or want to do to them. Many have never explored their own reaction to touch. Madalaine encourages us all to touch ourselves, caress our skin, try out new places (without genital touching, slightly to my relief. The genitals and intimate areas are off limits today).

There are soft gasps of joy as thirty-five women in a small, hot tent discover the tenderness and delicious sensations possible when they stroke the insides of their arms. Or their throats. Or let their own touch linger without judgement on the parts of themselves that women are taught to loathe. I caress my capacious inner thighs, thinking how often I have felt hate towards my wobblers in a culture that glorifies a thigh gap. Next, I lovingly stroke my bulging belly which has birthed two humans. Feeling not the usual toughness of the internal voice which has been taught self-disgust at this flabby shortcoming, but instead approaching my tummy and thighs with self-acceptance and gratitude for my sturdy, trusty body.

I find myself thinking that although the culture may tell me that I am a failure because I am not thin and toned, the reality is that I have a career, am loved, have two daughters, a husband of nearly three decades' standing and – pah! – I've managed all of that *with* fat thighs. So, the circumference of the tops of my legs is really *not* that important. Okay, I admit to my own conditioning. But believe me, that thought feels embarrassingly, deliciously, liberating!

Around me, young women speak of how sex for them has often been all about pleasuring a man, his needs, his satisfaction, his desire. About becoming an object for his gaze, his delectation, not about their own sexual pleasure. Several women with large breasts describe how their relationship with them has become warped because of the attention they garnered from a young age from men. They describe frantic attempts to cover them up. Or how they don't even think of their breasts as being part of them anymore because they have been so externally objectified for so long. I find myself relating to that. I remember being a girl in the sixth form of Westminster, a boys' public school in London where there were 800 boys and around 80 girls back in the 1980s.

No one called me Eleanor, they called me 'Jugs'. As a greeting, they'd go: 'Hello, Leftie, hello, Rightie … oh, hello, Eleanor.' As if I was an afterthought. Less important than my breasts.

It was not just at school that this would happen. Not as openly, sure, but I got so sick of men talking to my chest, not my eyes. In the yurt one woman talks about how her body had for so long been broken down into parts that people would comment on – nice legs, good tits, lovely hair – that she feels it doesn't really have much to do with her, the person. There is a rustle of agreement, a murmur of deep recognition. That is what objectification does; it makes our bodies not feel like our own, our physical home – but instead a commodity to be traded, inspected by men.

Some of the women weep, describing how their own relationships with their body have become warped and terrifying because of the memories of sexual abuse stored in their most intimate parts. They speak of how they had been violated by fathers or brothers, or friends of their parents; adults who were supposed to care for them. What is clear is that the legacy of that early abuse is shame and pain in private places that should have given them pleasure.

The wise leader of the workshop explains that one route back to a more positive relationship with their own pleasure, their own sexuality, is through self-touch. After all, if we are in charge, pleasuring ourselves, it is always safe, we can always stop. There is no other person involved who can hurt us. She explains that having gained sensory self-knowledge of ourselves we could then own it and share that insight with our lovers. The women talk about how good it feels to touch themselves slowly and softly. How pleasant it is to be gently stroked all over their bodies – not just the genitals or breasts beloved of men. Several of the women speak about how this experience is giving them confidence; they say they are going to go back to their partners and ask for what they really like, really want.

It was such a strange and unusual experience to be lying with thirty or so other women as they unpeeled themselves, explored their bodies (not the genitals, I repeat) but everywhere else. All of us sharing a safe and intimate space – helping and learning from each other's experiences and fears.

It made me think that if Queenagers ran the world such female-centred, sex-positive workshops would be mandatory in schools for teenage girls, and be widely available to all women. That if that were the case, how much more power, how much more joy women would have if we were all schooled from puberty to *expect* sensual pleasure. If we had it drummed into us that female satisfaction is a right. Were taught from the get-go that sex was about us, our orgasm, our pleasure, too – that sex is *not* just about pleasing men, or satisfying only them, but a mutual exchange, made better when women are equal partners, in charge of their desire and arousal. That we matter too.

We have been so conditioned, so programmed to be what men want rather than what we are. I am not blaming individual men for this but the way we have organised society – patriarchy – where men's needs come first and are serviced by women. Where female sexuality is primarily in service to men, not ourselves. I talk a lot about how the patriarchy values women primarily for youth, beauty and fertility; nowhere do we see that more than in how women are conditioned to view their role in sex. And nowhere is that more brutal or obvious than in pornography. If you want to see the male lens in action, click on Pornhub. Porn is shot from the male point of view – so that men feel they are there. They are the actor.

So where does that leave us and our sexuality as we age? Lost. The whole idea of Queenagers and sex is a kind of taboo topic. The very thought of oldies having sex is a horror show for many. But this is so not the reality. During the many sessions I have chaired on this subject with women from the Noon community, and in research we were part of with a female team who are creating a new vibrator for midlife women, I've seen that sex goes on being a very important and active part of older women's lives. Whether that is about taking the time for active and indulgent shame-free self-pleasure, or sex with a partner.

Of course, it is not all swinging from the chandeliers. I also hear about many couples who live kind of parallel but not interconnected lives, who go through the motions of marriage but no longer share a bedroom. In many marriages, after several decades sexual intimacy is no longer part of the equation. I understand that. But I am writing this because it doesn't have to be like that; it is not the whole picture.

I recently conducted a survey of the women in my community, asking them to describe what sex was like for them in their fifties and beyond. These are just some of the things they wrote: 'Sex is warmth, orange, deep and safe.' 'I feel a deep connection with my husband; we have been together so long.' 'It is way more passionate and less inhibited than when we were younger.' 'Sex now is loving, calm, natural.' 'Dreamy tingling.' 'Fading but with brilliant spots of colour.' 'Passionate, mind-blowing, erotic, dirty and surprising.' 'Fantastic, unbelievably good.' 'I feel more confident and desirable.' 'Sex for me now is exciting, overwhelming – warm happy.' One of my favourites was a woman who said, 'I find sex now is gentler, goes on for longer and is sometimes surprisingly intense with rainbow leg orgasms.'

Rainbow leg orgasms? Nope, me neither!

But what this does show, I think, is that sexual chemistry, passion and intimacy really can be alive and well, even after so many decades. Amanda's story which follows is typical of what I hear from my Queenagers, but which we never, or rarely, hear in the mainstream.

Amanda is fifty-six and says she has always liked sex and that in her life she has been lucky to have many sexual partners. 'But I can honestly put my hand on my heart and say I have never had sex as good as the sex I have now in my late fifties.' Her orgasms last longer and are more intense; she experiences a kind of synaesthesia where all her senses merge – like seeing sound, hearing colour. Sometimes she says she leaves her body completely as 'if I am floating around with my husband in a completely different dimension'. She says she never felt this way when she was younger but that, with the passing of the two decades they have been together, they now know each other so well and are so uninhibited around each other and their bodies that they have gone way beyond self-consciousness or worrying about wobbly bits or whether they are doing it right.

'Now when we make love there is just a total sense of union, of playfulness – of everything being allowed and acceptable. It is just a sense of wholeness, of love and intimacy, but also being fully known. It is beautiful, unlike anything I have ever known before. A power that is unapologetic and in union with sexuality.'

We talked about what has made the difference between how sex feels now compared to when she was younger. She says that the difference is trust, an intimate trust built up over twenty-five years of loving each other. 'We have always had a strong physical chemistry, but since our children have left home and since my menopause, sex has become different, more intense, more abandoned. It sounds a bit unfeminist, but I think that in the autumn of my life, the youth of old age, I have finally learnt how to truly receive. To really think about that, to wait and let him come inside me in increments rather than rushing, to engage my vaginal muscles to encourage that entry. To wait. To take pleasure in submission and the art of submission. That is the difference.'

She says that these were not things she had ever thought about or known about when she was younger, but that this new openness to receptivity and a more engaged sense of being entirely there in the moment are what have made the difference. 'My sex life is transformed. Even my idea of what sex is, is different. I've learnt to embrace patience; I have a new sense of setting my body to a receive setting. The pleasure in that and in the idea of submission is a new thing for me. It's not something I have read about anywhere; it is something I have found for myself. But it has definitely come from being less in a hurry. Less grasping, more prepared to wait and have it come to me. Maybe it is because I am more relaxed, more truly in the moment, totally there. Also maybe more confident. My orgasms have never been more pleasurable or intense.'

It is a great myth that only young bodies can have great sex. I want everyone to know about this autumn flowering, how, as we age, our bodies can become more primed for pleasure, more able to give and receive rapture than they have ever been.

I tried out Amanda's insights on a group of my closest friends. There was a great sense of recognition. A few giggles and then admissions that they too were having better sex in their fifties than they had ever had before. They all agreed with what Amanda had told me. One friend said: 'My body is now more primed for pleasure, more able to give and receive rapture than it has ever been. I know that now we have the house to ourselves I feel freer. Our lovemaking can last for over an hour. It can be a slow burn, long lingering caresses. Stroking each other all over our bodies. We light candles, we listen to music, we take our time. We know we will not be disturbed.'

But she added that more than this sense of a slow build and privacy after twenty years of raising children is what has changed inside her own head, inside her own body. 'When I was younger, often when we had sex I was tired, or busy, or running through my to-do list or thinking about what I might wear the next day to a meeting. Maybe I was eager to get it done so I could sleep – or I was distracted by the children downstairs. But in retrospect I think I was too eager to get to the climax and I don't think I had realised what my true role in getting there was. I think maybe I took too much responsibility; I was grasping after it rather than waiting for it to come to me. I've discovered sweet pleasure in the waiting, in the passivity; it is not something that I had ever explored before. But it is as if I have come into my full power as a woman and the sex feels more than just bodies, like a truly spiritual union, a oneness. And physically the orgasms are much more powerful and last longer.'

We hear a lot about how long-term relationships inevitably go sexually stale. I know that is true of some couples, and I do have friends for whom menopause and post-menopause and some vaginal dryness have meant that sex has become painful. I'm happy to report that they say that using a good lubricant, or 'lube', can work miracles.

There are so many horror stories out there about wrinkled old women and how we are crones who don't want sex. I don't think that is true; it is what society has conditioned us to believe. I also come across some older men (often no oil paintings themselves) who speak about older women as if they are repugnant, revolting, as if women have sell-by dates – and yet somehow they don't! (I sometimes wonder if these men have actually looked at themselves in a mirror in the last ten years. How they can be paunchy and yet judge women who dare not to be pencils is beyond me.) I just know that is not the whole story – both from talking to male friends of my own age who say how they still fancy their wives of the same age and from talking to my own friends. Many of my single Queenager friends are now dating younger men whom they find very sexually satisfying and who also recognise the power of the Autumn Queen in the bedroom.

Maybe that is what some older men of the dinosaur mentality are afraid of … mature women in touch with their own sexuality and desires. Not in thrall to the old male gaze. But if we are talking about conditioning and how we are programmed to feel, just because we may have a few wrinkles doesn't mean we stop being sexual beings. My cousin got remarried in her eighties and had a very satisfying sex life. We don't have to believe the gendered-ageist hype out there which tells us that old women are dried-up husks. Nor do we have to be sexually active as we age if we don't want to be. But it can be very, very good! Sex can get much better as we age. Surely that is something to look forward to. I wish more women knew that.

Secret: Sex gets better with age. I have more intense orgasms than I ever did when I was younger, probably because I know my husband and my body so well and I am no longer self-conscious. I also feel a connection to something bigger, more existential; a sense of surrender, of giving and receiving pleasure in a way I didn't as a young woman. So, make the most of being an Autumn Queen! Whether that's with a partner or on your own. Prioritise pleasure – after all, we only live once.

Reprogramming – you are enough

I am at a tiny women's festival deep in the English countryside. When I open the flap of my tent the park is full of mist; I can hardly see the trees on the opposite side of the valley.

Two hours later and the sun is bright, a late flowering of summer after a chilly August. I am moving and stomping in the middle of a huge field, surrounded, at a distance, by other women dancing to their own rhythm, following their own wave. Clamped to my ears are a pair of headphones streaming tunes for my Ecstatic Dance session. If I remove them, all is quiet, except for birdsong and the odd whoop of delight. When I replace them, I am back on the virtual dancefloor, in the snare of the DJ whose commanding sound is bidding me to move, to march, to stomp, to wave my arms, bend over and salute the ground, gyrate with joy.

I am always an enthusiastic dancer but this dancing is different. Grooving in broad daylight in the middle of a deer park, I am freed from any external – male – gaze. For maybe the first time in my life, or certainly for the first time since I was a child, I am moving and dancing only for myself; following whatever impulse takes me in a gush of what feels like intense freedom.

There is no one watching me. I move because I want to, I allow my body to do whatever it feels. I do not need to be sexy, or move my limbs to look attractive in the way that I now realise I subconsciously always have – to greater or lesser degrees – in a nightclub or at a party.

I don't slip into my normal hip-swinging shimmy, perfected over so many years of being on show. Nope. Instead, this morning I march, arms swinging to the beat up and down the field. I stamp my feet. I find myself making horizontal and vertical lines, I jump up and down on the spot for the sheer hell of it, holding my bouncing breasts so they are not uncomfortable (not my usual look at a party, I assure you). I skip like I did as a kid. I put my head between my knees and whizz my arms round like helicopter blades. I stand still and feel the soft grass under my feet and the soil beneath that. I am in my body. Dancing with myself. Free and happy.

Around me women of all ages, races, shapes and sizes are doing exactly what they feel in this moment. Many strip down to their knickers, breasts open to the air and the trees, embracing the liberation of sunlight on skin, the removal of bras and constriction. Some wander off into the woods, or find a special tree to dance with. In this safe space the only eyes on us are our own, and we are all doing it too, or wild creatures (who probably think we're bonkers). Dancing with abandon feels like a rare moment of no judgement, no pressure, no critical gaze (even my internal one is switched off).

It is heady. Hard even to know what to do with such freedom. One woman lies down on the dewy grass and rubs her breasts and stomach into the earth. Others waggle their tits at the woods. The music speeds up and slows down; and as it changes I inhabit many moods and aspects of myself. Purposeful, whimsical, still, whirling dervish – anything I like. In the two hours I spend dancing in this glorious green expanse, with lime, beech and oak trees creating a protective ring around the edges, I am entirely present, gloriously me. Free.

It is a revelation.

The night before, I lay on the ground in a red Rajasthani tent, while an artist played crystal bowls and gongs and sang, creating a meditational bubble of sacred sound all around me. Inside the cacophony I found a moment or two of total stillness. Following the sound, I melted so far into the ground that I felt I was no longer lying on the surface of the earth but had been absorbed into Gaia's crust; waves of fully grown barley and wheat undulated across the top of my belly. I was a hillock, a bit of sod, part of Mother Earth, plants and trees growing out of and through me. The sense deepened and it was as if rivers were flowing and waves crashing deep inside of me; that I was simultaneously everything and nothing. My body contained the universe, was a part of the earth – it was the strangest sensation.

I have had yoga and meditation teachers tell me so often to 'ground' myself, to think of coils going from my pelvis down into the earth. To feel connected to it, to feel the earth's energy, its gravity pulling me to it. Of course, I tried to do what they asked. But I have never felt 'embodied' in the ground before, literally part of it, as if I had become just a clod of earth. A rock. And before you ask, no, I hadn't taken any mushrooms, or anything else for that matter; the entire festival was stimulant-free. I was just absorbing this magical soundscape and sinking and sinking down, so relaxed and present and warm that the 'I' of me just dissolved. While taking psilocybin in Jamaica I have felt like I was a bit of soil, suffused with green light of growing energy; I could sense microbes and worms around me, and roots. But this was different. I was it, there was no separation.

The whole three days at the women's festival felt like a reprogramming. Maybe it was so many hours lying on the ground, or the presence of so many like-minded women, but it was as if a whole section of my brain – which is usually on high alert for risk – was deactivated. As if I could just be me. I think that is the journey we are on with our Queenager bodies. Moving away from them being considered external assets, sexualised 'bits' for others to comment on or enjoy; or from the thinness or otherwise of our bodies being something to be concerned about; or from needing to force them into an externally dictated shape. Midlife for me has meant feeling more loving towards my body, feeling fond of my wrinkly hands which have held my babies and written so many words. Feeling joy in my sturdy legs which have carried me faithfully for half a century. Feeling a sense of release and freedom from the prescriptions of stupid glossy magazines which are just trying to make women buy stuff. And, most of all, feeling grounded, present, truly embodied inside my own precious frame. Health scares, our own and those of others, force us to see that just being here, in a body that still works in midlife and beyond, is a gift. That being able to age is a privilege. After a lifetime of battle, I feel like I have put down my weapons and can finally inhabit and feel joy inside my own skin. Maybe you can too.

Secret: The key to deep body acceptance is that grounding sense that we are Gaians, part of Mother Earth, lucky to be here for this brief time. That we in our physicality are miracles, spiritual beings having an earthly experience which is all about being in this flesh. That rather than critiquing our vessel, we should celebrate and enjoy it. It is the only home we ever have.

PART SIX

SPIRITUALITY

The part of my story that feels most private, that has remained most hidden, is my journey into more spiritual realms. My years as a cynical hack, an editor whose job it was to weigh evidence, to test truths, found the very idea of 'spirit' anathema. I was brought up a strict atheist; our family religion was No Religion. And my education was firmly Enlightenment-based: *cogito, ergo sum* – I think, therefore I am. Oxford University taught me to value intellect over feeling, reasoning over intuition. Twenty-five years at a newspaper only reinforced that.

Yet, to shapeshift into my Queenager self, I have had to discover new ways of knowing, of being. I used to feel like my body was extraneous except as a way to carry my brain around. Now I am more in tune with it; I've learnt to listen to its tingles, or prickles, as good barometers of big truth or warnings. Some would describe that as tuning in to my intuition, that embodied sense of knowing; we are, after all, animals.

If you'd asked me before if I was a spiritual person I would have scoffed. Now I would say yes, of course. When I meditate, I am aware of tapping into a field, a flickering sense of colour, of connection inside my eyelids. It has become an essential part of my day to tune in to that alongside a greater appreciation of the connectedness of all things and the natural world. This is the story of my journey into other realms, other ways of being – of inhabiting stillness, exploring the great glory and gift of being alive.

The trip that changed my life

Now, if I am really honest, the seeds of the new me were sown before I left my big job. It was while I was still the editor of the *Sunday Times* magazine, on the week of my forty-ninth birthday, that I went to take magic mushrooms on a supervised psilocybin retreat in Jamaica. I'd gone because my friend and fellow journalist Decca had PTSD – post-traumatic stress disorder. Her husband had drowned in front of her and her two young sons, five years before (she wrote a brilliant book about it called *All at Sea*, if you'd like to know more). In the following years she had once more taken up her glittering career as the best interviewer on Fleet Street and had come to work for me. As a single mother, she had soldiered on, survived breast cancer – she was diagnosed a year after her husband drowned – as well as the bereavement (an epic midlife collision), but when she came to tell me that she wanted to go on the mushroom retreat and write about it, she admitted that, although functional, the tumultuous events of the preceding years had left her feeling numb. She couldn't feel all the terrible stuff – but she couldn't feel any of the good bits either; not joy when her kids hugged her, or happiness when surrounded by friends.

We'd both read Michael Pollan's book *How to Change Your Mind* about psychedelics and particularly the efficacy of magic mushrooms (psilocybin) to help cure depression and PTSD. Pollan describes how the psilocybin acts like a new fall of snow on a deeply grooved slope, smoothing over the old ruts so the mind can make fresh tracks

– particularly useful when we have got stuck in a loop of negative ruminative thoughts we can't escape.

Decca had found a retreat in Jamaica where shrooms could be taken legally (Jamaica never got round to banning them) and she wanted to try psilocybin in this therapeutic setting and write about it for the magazine I then edited. I thought it was a great story and immediately said yes – but with one proviso: if she was going, I said, I was going with her. I justified that decision by saying that others on the retreat might not want to be written about so I could be her 'friend' if she needed colour, and by saying I had a duty of care towards her as her editor if she was going to do something so dangerous. But that wasn't the real reason I went.

I didn't know then why I was so adamant about joining her. Now I would say that my 'awakened self' called to me knowing that that fateful trip (sorry) was going to mark the beginning of my new life (and an amazing and life-defining new friendship). At the time I was rather confused at my massive enthusiasm to go; back then Decca and I were boss and journalist, we liked each other but we weren't that close. I can just remember feeling an overwhelming sense that I had to go: as if the deepest part of me was yelling, 'Yes! This! Now! Don't ask why, just do it!'

I'd never thought about taking magic mushrooms before; indeed, at university I'd always been scared of acid and all hallucinogens, having grown up on apocalyptic tales of people jumping out of windows while tripping because they thought they could fly. Like most Queenagers of my generation, I'd taken ecstasy as part of the rave scene in my late teens and smoked some pot. But hallucinogens were in my drug Room 101, along with heroin. 'Just Say No' was what we were taught. I'd always been fine with that.

But on the day when Decca told me about Jamaica, something deep in my soul screamed: 'Yes. This.' I was quite determined that I was going – even though it felt terrifying and I didn't know why I wanted to go (and my husband thought I was nuts and I thought I might *go* nuts). But the truth is, that trip truly changed my life.

Let me set the scene. The retreat took place in an old colonial house on a steep slope above the sea on Jamaica's southern coast. Picture an idyllic tropical garden; palm trees and hummingbirds, bougainvillea and rainbow-coloured flowers. The place buzzed with life and beauty. On the retreat the mantra was 'set and setting'. 'Setting' means creating a totally safe environment. No surprises, no responsibilities. A phalanx of trusty trip sitters (like babysitters, but for people who are off their heads) are always around so that no one gets hurt and if you are frightened there is someone *compos mentis* and reassuring to chat to. The dose is carefully calculated and takes the form of mushrooms in powdered form in capsules (they look like vitamins). Before each trip there is a guided meditation to 'set' the mood and intention for that day's experience. During the first we were told to imagine bright white light above our heads, a feeling of safety, a place we could return to if things took a dark turn. On the second, to envision our younger selves and to gather them up and take them with us on the journey. The 'set' done and the mushrooms taken, we retreatants retired to a sunlounger in the shade with a musical playlist to go wherever the mushrooms led.

We did three trips during the week. My moment of true epiphany happened on the last one. We sat in a circle, above the sea, azure waves breaking on the rocks below, palm fronds brushing the roof of the domed meditation pavilion. 'Take anything you no longer need in your life and throw it off a cliff, or blow it up …' said the soothing voice of one of the trip facilitators. Without any thought, I found myself putting my whole career at the media group that had been my life for the past two decades into a box and blowing it up with a golden beam from my heart. I exploded it all. All my ambitions, all the work I had put into being an editor. It fell away.

And I felt amazing. Light as air. Relieved. Unburdened. It wasn't done consciously; I hadn't even known I wanted to get out. I blew it all up entirely spontaneously, it just felt right in that moment. Essential even.

But when I told Decca what I had done, she was not delighted. 'You

can't blow up your whole career at the paper,' she said. 'You're my boss!
I need you!'

I laughed.

'Sorry, mate, I just did.'

Twenty minutes or so after that meditation, my final trip began.
I had taken 8 grams of psilocybin. A hero dose. No micro-dosing here!
During the first two trips I had felt ecstatic, had danced around filled
with energy (on the second one I'd thought I was a jack-in-the-box; for
six hours I was a carefree child, laughing and naughty, jumping around).

This time I felt heavy and had to lie down. I felt a deep need for
solitude, for peace, to be away from everyone, even Decca.

I retreated to a calm, quiet spot under a palm tree beyond a hedge
beside a pool above the sea and put Bob Marley's song 'One Love' on
repeat on the stereo. I lay down and the heaviness lifted instantly. Above
me, the green leaves played against the blue sky, moving so slowly it
felt like time had stopped, like I could fall between the gaps between
the seconds, like I was in one eternal moment. I closed my eyes and
the insides of my lids were flooded with golden light; I felt like I was
floating in a bowl of cream, immersed in a magical reviving elixir.
The bit that was me, Eleanor, separate, distinct from other beings, had
entirely dissolved into the golden light. I had no idea where I ended and
the golden liquid began – but it didn't matter. It was all good. I realised
that there was no division, that I was everything, that everything was
inside me. It was all one. All light, all energy. All pulsing life.

I had a strong sense that day of being plugged into a cosmic recharger
– of being rebooted, re-energised by the universe. Plugged in and
revved up for a whole new era, a whole new life and mission. It was
transformational. I was shown the connectedness of everything. How
all humans, and animals and plants, are linked together through a web
of interconnected and intermeshed, throbbing life. That there is no
separation, only oneness. That we are all built from the same golden
light; that it is life and is everywhere and in everything around us.

Animating all. I lay there for at least forty-five minutes, totally content. Bob playing in the background. Blissed out.

When I was able to start moving again, I floated in a pool, drifting up and down with my breath, not knowing where my body stopped and the water began. It was all one. I felt perfectly happy. Afterwards I stood dazed and joyous on a ledge overlooking the sea, feeling and conducting all the energy I could sense in my heightened state in the breeze and air around me. As the sun set, I sat next to Decca looking out over the turquoise sea as the song 'Don't Worry, Be Happy' played, as if by magic. It was a random playlist but suddenly it boomed out, at the perfect moment. It felt like everything was in flow, all was unfolding exactly as it was supposed to be. That everything was indeed perfect.

We sat together and held hands. Decca was smiling, tears running down her cheeks, weeping with relief that she could *feel* again. That the numb dam had broken. (The piece she wrote about that experience was nominated as the best long article of 2020 by the BBC.)

We vowed that, from then on, we would say yes to joy.

It felt that simple.

I committed that day to a new path for myself; and to help others tread that path too. It was in my 'golden moment' when I conceived the idea for Noon, realised that a total shift, a transformation in world-view in midlife was possible. That we really could find and become different versions of ourselves even on the cusp of our fifth decade or beyond. The golden light had shown me the way. I decided that talking about that, enacting it, helping women make that change, that shift into being and feeling something new, was what I wanted to do. I know it sounds crazy but I felt on some very deep level as if I'd finally found my thing, my calling. My true purpose. It was a profound moment of becoming ... or, rather, as I was to discover subsequently, the beginning of my becoming.

Of course, three months later when I was made redundant (a massive shock, although in some way I had called it in) and my whole life at the paper truly imploded, it didn't feel wonderful at all. I was in freefall.

But even in those darkest moments, when I meditated (which I started to do every day when I was ill with Covid at the beginning of lockdown) I discovered I could find my way back to that sense of golden light, of connection with all things. It was why, in my time of maximum darkness, the phrase 'Golden light. Golden light.' became my mantra. That feeling of reconnection, of oneness, was truly my light in the darkness, the beacon that guided me through all the doubts and tribulations that were to come. At some deep level I was glad. I was free. I was becoming a different version of me. The experience of that golden trip helped me through the dark days after my redundancy. The light in the darkness.

Denise, the woman leading the meditation that day in Jamaica who encouraged me to throw away everything that no longer served me, was, although I hadn't yet coined the term, a fellow Queenager. She was there because, at sixty, she had decided she was sick of playing it small; she left her secure job as a psychiatric social worker in the US, locked her possessions into storage and set off.

After the retreat, she took me to the little house by the sea where she was living in a tiny room with one suitcase: like a student traveller. I thought it looked a bit spartan, a bit sad. She disagreed. 'Not having any stuff makes me feel free,' she said. When I asked how she'd wound up there, she said she often wondered the same thing herself. It made me ponder that idea of the 'awakened self': was the Denise who rose at dawn, talked to dragonflies and did yoga on the Jamaican coast the same woman who had been a therapist back on the East Coast in the US? Had this version of her, or indeed my new version of me, or your potential version of yourself, been latent all along, living inside her, or me, or you? Denise described years of loss – the death of her husband, her brother; her mother's descent into dementia and her children leaving the nest – as the layers unpeeling. 'Losing all of them had left me so unmoored that it was easier to set sail,' she said.

Like me and Decca, Denise had set off for the psilocybin retreat

because of Pollan's book; as a psychologist she was convinced that
psychedelic-assisted treatment was the future and wanted to be part of it.
'The mushroom reached into my cells and wrung out decades' worth of
grief, pain, shame and regret,' Denise said of that first retreat. 'I howled
and wept, great rivers of snot running down my face. I recounted my
story of loss to a facilitator whose tears glittered like diamonds, whose
tattoo seemed to weep blood. I shook my fists at the heavens and begged:
"A little help here!" A star-glistened staircase descended from the skies.
When I spoke of grief, my feet seemed to sink into mud and the branches
of the almond tree grew gnarly and reached for me menacingly. When
I spoke of gratitude, the same tree burst into blossom. Most importantly,
I experienced a deep self-cherishing. I acknowledged all I had lost and
overcome, and, for the first time ever, realised what a badass I was.'

I love that. That badass Queenager moment of realising what we
can do, be, become.

Of course, as with my own journey that moment of revelation is
followed by making the dream a reality. I have always been interested in
the granularity of the path, how we make the decision to change, what
that looks like in terms of the everyday, the steps taken, the pebbles that
we follow on the route to our destination. For Denise, too, the lightbulb
moment was followed by insecurity and doubt. Friends thought she was
mad to be giving up a secure job as a therapist, a pension, her lovely
home, her poetry club and carefully constructed life. But her son was
enthusiastic and told her to listen to 'her soul's shout' and reminded her
she wouldn't actually want the lives any of the naysayers were leading.

So Denise took the plunge. Her first weeks were idyllic – all fresh
honey from backyard beehives, journalling while sipping Blue Mountain
coffee, swimming at dawn in turquoise waters. Inevitably, though, it
wasn't all plain sailing. The twelve-hour days tending to guests on
mushroom retreats left her semi-comatose with exhaustion. 'I was by
far the oldest member of the team and was worried about being able to
keep up. We cycled through a variety of other retreat facilitators – some

I liked; some made me prickly. I felt like Wendy tending to Peter Pan's Lost Boys. It certainly wasn't all lounging in a hammock with a Red Stripe.' Some days she was homesick and lonely, and particularly missed spending time with women her own age, but there was something liberating about travelling so light. 'I had space, finally, to examine the early conditioning from teachers/preachers/parents which had shaped who I had become. Like an archaeologist at a dig, I sifted through my life. What artefacts were gems? What needed to go?'

This is the job for all of us in midlife. Denise says that she felt 'the same elation she had when she set out for college' forty years earlier. In Jamaica, she was filled with what the German poet Rilke described as 'living my life in widening circles' and a strong sense that she is not done with her changes.

Looking back now, it seems too apt that a fellow Queenager should have been the one to show me the way to my next chapter. That it was her wise words, and entreaty to shed that which I didn't even consciously know I had to lose, that put me on this new path. I suppose the moral of this tale is, when an opportunity arises, to listen keenly to your body's deep intuitive response, even if it seems logically weird and not the kind of thing you would usually do. A couple of times in my life I have felt that pull. When I met my husband Derek in India – I just knew I had found my soulmate. And when Decca said she was going to Jamaica and my soul just screamed, 'YES!'

See a wise woman – she helped me. I'm sure her words will help you.

Secret: There are times in our lives when we are called, when the route to our new self and what we might become is opened to us. In retrospect it is clear. At the time it just feels like a bizarre but incredibly strong pull towards something new or random. My advice is to take it – grab it with both hands. Jump. And be on the lookout for it. Don't quash it or push it away. Listen for the call of your 'awakened' self.

We belong in nature

The mushroom retreat was just the beginning of my midlife spiritual journey. It acted as a bit of a jump-start, opening a window to other realms of my mind. Other possibilities. I became a bit of a seeker. I wanted to see if I could find that golden place of connection without the psychedelics. After I left the paper, still in the doldrums, I joined a retreat in Yorkshire. I knew no one; had no pal to anchor me, wasn't there as a journalist. There was no escaping it. I was there to work on myself.

Driving up to Skipton, I felt unmoored. Not sure what on earth I was doing. I had arrived a day late and was taken to join the group who were standing in the middle of a field surrounded by sheep. A woman with kind eyes and a strong Yorkshire accent told us to close our eyes and 'feel the breeze'. She told us to be aware of what our senses were picking up. A sheep going *baaa*. The smell of the grass. She seemed very sure. I remember smelling sheep shit and hearing a lorry changing gear on the road. This was after the mushroom retreat, but I was in the midst of rejection and redundancy – my journalistic cynicism was turned up to maximum.

Then she led us into the nearby wood. The instruction? 'Just be.' FFS, I thought. That meant spending an hour pottering about – she called it 'forest bathing'; apparently it is big in Japan. Trees give off chemicals that not only allow them to communicate with each other but which calm our nervous systems, she explained. It didn't seem to be working on me. My brain was going at a thousand miles an hour. I kept reaching for my phone, for distraction. It and I were umbilically attached, but I had had to hand it in on arrival at the retreat. It felt weird to be so untethered. Like a child without its dummy. Or a smoker without cigarettes. I literally didn't know how I would get through the next sixty minutes. I mooched about and tried to make what-the-hell-*is*-this faces at some of the other women. I'm a natural rebel, the naughty one in the group; I was looking for a partner in crime. But they all avoided my gaze. One woman was lovingly holding the tendrils of a willow tree. Others were hugging trunks, or looking around, rapt. I wasn't going to find any fellow cynics here.

Then I noticed the stream – and realised I was wearing my wellies. Hah! I remembered how, when I was a kid, I would spend hours walking up and down the stream near our house. Kicking rocks, making dams, pottering. I hadn't done that for years. The idea of water was more appealing than the wintry woods so I went in. I slithered down a bank and sloshed about. The water felt cool running over my boots. I watched the ripples and the eddies and even built a dam out of some rotten wood to create a larger pool. A shaft of sunlight glittered. I leant against a tree and found myself crying a bit into its solidness. The trunk felt comforting, like the arms of my husband. I stretched out against it and wrapped my arms around its trunk; I looked up to where branches turned into twigs. Up there a few last leaves, high overhead, danced with the wind and the sky. Below I could feel the water and rocks under the soles of my feet. The whistle blew. I realised the hour had passed surprisingly swiftly.

The woman – Liz – brewed tea on a fire she had made in a clearing. There was moss of iridescent green. We sat on logs and she served the hot liquid in delicate Japanese porcelain cups, handing them to each of us with ceremony. With reverence. I could feel her calmness, her ease in the wood and this moment.

She touched me.

Liz hadn't always been a forest guru. Nine years before, she had been a solicitor in a top London law firm. Like many of us, Liz thought she was ticking all the boxes society asked of her. She had the big City job, designer clothes, a good salary, but it never felt like it was enough. 'I don't ever recall feeling I belonged. In truth, I never felt good enough. I was known for my good humour, the ever-smiling team member, the one who was great at networking events. I never revealed my true self: inside, I felt desperately lonely, sad and incompetent.'

Her parents had been workaholics and 'this pattern of behaviour became my survival mechanism. I worked at the weekends, often the only person in the office. I worked late nights and early mornings, anything to avoid my feelings. And although I didn't know it at the time, I worked to please others.' The incessant workload, the long hours, the stress, the anxiety, would often become too much. Alcohol increasingly became her crutch. After-work drinks on a Friday would frequently turn into all-night binge-drinking sessions and, on sobering up, she would despise herself and feel overwhelmed with shame. Knowing something had to change, she signed up to the Hoffman Process, a seven-day residential course with the tagline 'when you're serious about change'.

A month later, she left her job and put her flat on the market.

She studied mindfulness and then travelled to Nepal and walked the Himalayas. She was so moved by the beauty of the mountains that she realised her essence, her spirit, 'needed to be in nature, that that was going to be a massive part of my new life'. Following a well-trodden spiritual path, she went from Nepal to the holy city of Varanasi in India and then on to Rishikesh.

Although she didn't know it at the time, Liz was on a classic Indian path called Vanaprastha. I found out about it during a circle I ran for Indian Queenagers. It's a twenty-five-year phase meaning 'retiring to the forest', which usually happens between the ages of fifty and seventy-four, when traditionally elders go into nature to discover wisdom. Vanaprastha is part of four Hindu cycles of life: student; householder;

hermit/forest dweller; wandering ascetic or holy man (or woman!).
This Hindu version of what Avivah would call Q3 is about gradually
withdrawing from the world to live a more spiritual and solitary life at
one with nature. It reflects a profound shift from being focused on the
material pursuits of wealth and pleasure and family to looking inward,
towards self-realisation and, ultimately, unity with the natural world
and the divine. Similarly to Liz, Chitra, one of the Indian Queenagers
I interviewed, talked of midlife for her being about noticing animals,
birds and natural patterns, being outside more, becoming more tuned
in. 'I had to remind myself not to work all the time. We live our lives
in cycles, transitions, changing our colours; it is how the natural world
works too. We can't keep extracting from ourselves without giving back
and expect we will just regenerate, that there will be an endless well
to draw from. We need some fallow, wallowing time to do some inner
searching. Like Buddha who wandered for fourteen years asking what
is the purpose? Why am I here, what am I doing?'

During Liz's fallow period in India she delved deep into herself,
exploring the pain of loneliness, the pain of feeling the constant pres-
sure to be pleasing others, the pain of continually striving and never
feeling good enough. These are all subjects that are now very familiar
to me from listening to so many Queenagers in our Noon Circles, and
what I have learnt from sitting with all these wounds is that they do not
stem from our own unique, pathetic weaknesses – they are systemic.
We women have been programmed by our society, our culture, to feel
like this, to act like this, to put everyone else's needs and wants ahead
of our own. But like me and so many others while working through
these griefs, Liz cried and cried and cried. But she ultimately found
that releasing the anguish was liberating.

When she returned to England she remembered a conversation she'd
had on her travels about forest bathing and applied to do the six-month
training programme. It blended mindfulness with her new-found love
of Mother Nature, honed during her daily walks in the mountains and

now essential to her peace of mind. Forest bathing in its simplest form is taking a slow walk in a natural environment but, as a practice, it is so much more. On a forest-bathing walk, we take time out from our everyday lives and, with nature as a mirror, we often meet aspects of ourselves that we haven't noticed in a long time. When I tried it, I found that childish playfulness in the water and a deep sense of support and succour in my hug with a tree. Spending time with nowhere to go, no focus except just being with trees, in the river, in nature, allows us to slow down, rediscover our relationship with the natural world and, best of all, it is entirely instinctive – as I found, sploshing around in that stream in my wellies.

For the past four years, Liz has been teaching forest bathing. In reconnecting people with nature and helping them to slow down and just be, she says she has found her calling. 'When I walked out of the London office that day I took a huge leap of faith. I haven't ever regretted it. There are still aspects of my life that are not "perfect" but now I feel every day is to be lived, not just endured, and I love it.'

By that Liz means she has learnt how to find joy in simple things. She often sends me videos of her dancing to power ballads high in the Yorkshire Dales, or sitting in a drumming circle teaching visitors to throw off their self-consciousness and feel the great freedom and rhythm that comes from hitting a drum. Whether it is lighting fires (a real Liz passion) or spreading hilarity with her infectious giggle, Liz has used nature to reconnect with that sense of lightness at just being in the world. Something that had got crushed under the pressures of society's demands and expectations.

Secret: It is never too late to start living a life that you love. Have the confidence to trust your instincts – if you are unhappy and things aren't going right, maybe it's time to turn left. And the ancient Hindu tradition of spending some time wallowing and fallowing close to nature is a great place to start.

Metamorphosis

It is one of those days in autumn that feels like spring. The sun is optimistically bright after a tempestuous rainstorm last night, the sky, trees and clouds appear washed clean. I feel the pond calling and when I get there it is decorated with bowers of leaves and flowers for the equinox, and the water is so green and sparkly it looks like tinsel. The air temperature is 13 degrees but the water is 18 – the heat comes off the surface as patches of mist which look like breath; like the pond is alive and breathing.

The magic here today is contagious. The women swim wreathed in smiles, hair backlit.

Usually I am content to swim on the surface, luxuriating in the expanse of sky above and the trees around. But this morning I dive down repeatedly, imagining I am a seal, opening my eyes underwater as I return to the surface, watching as the murky yellow-brown of the water turns gold then blue as I see the sky above.

I wonder where my friend the heron is, I haven't seen him for a couple of days; and, as if summoned by my thoughts, he is suddenly there, looming above me, wings wide, larger than a person. I watch as he tries to land in the green and gold foliage of a silver birch. But the branch is too weak to hold him and he slips back and flaps right over my head again, huge and menacing, before perching high in an oak tree behind me.

As I swim and dive, marvelling at the pond's breath and all the living creatures around me, I wonder at the magic of this place, think about how, for all these years, it has been here but I was too busy to partake of it, too blind to see it, unattuned to the nature which now feels acutely necessary to me as a daily fix. In the pond life pulses around me, captures me in the moment, the feeling, the water, the now.

What is it about nature that creeps up on us at this point in our life – why do the birds seem to sing louder, the roses bloom more abundantly, the leaves throb? It is linked, I think, to the stripping away of layers. Dismantling the carapace, the armour, that, like a soul-callous, grew over the years I spent being a square peg in a round hole, constantly overriding my own instincts in order to fit with the demands of the organisation. I was so focused on attuning myself to others' wants and needs I'd entirely stopped listening to my true self.

The stripping away of the armour began with the psilocybin retreat; but the process has been ongoing.

One of the most powerful tools for me on this journey has been taking part in Constellations. Invented by German therapist Bert Hellinger in the 1990s and also known as Family Constellations, they are a way of exploring the beliefs we've inherited that keep us imprisoned, that lurk in our subconscious and get in our way. Using a constellation, a circle of people who act out different aspects of the problem to be explored, the process brings hidden beliefs to light so that they can be questioned, released and overwritten. It is hard to explain because it acts on a different, maybe deeper, level than our rational, Enlightenment, brain. The process is all about exploring other ways of knowing. It sounds whacky, I know. All I can say is, try it. It works.

It begins with tuning in to your intuition. A starter question could be something as simple as: Do you like cats or dogs? Or both, or neither. Whatever the answer, the group is split into different parts of the room according to what they feel about it. There is no right or wrong, just where *you* want to be, where feels right. Some were big dog lovers, some love cats, some both. Me? Neither particularly, I am allergic to both!

Next I am put in a group with two other women, Rachel and Jane. Rachel volunteers to go first; she will be the focus of the constellation. Three pieces of paper are placed on the ground in a line. The first represents the person we are now; Rachel stands here. The second represents our future self, the person we would like to be. Jane takes this position. Between Rachel and Jane is the third piece of paper – this represents everything that is stopping Rachel from becoming the person she would like to be. They stand gazing at one another, looking across a chasm that represents the roadblocks in Rachel's life. My job is to hold space, just to stand watching and tuning in to the two of them. And doing this, concentrating intently on Rachel while she contemplates the things that are blocking her from becoming the person she would like to be, I have a truly new – and very weird – experience.

First, I feel shaky and tearful. Then, suddenly, into my mind, like an incoming fax transmission, comes a black-and-white image, clear like a photograph or an X-ray. It is a woman I have never seen before, with platinum blonde hair and a short fringe. I look up and see that Rachel, the one doing the exercise, is weeping uncontrollably. I tell her about the weird picture in my head. 'Oh, that's my friend Melly,' she says, smiling through her sobs. Melly, she explains, died of cancer a few years ago but had been the woman who rescued Rachel from a terrible situation – the one she is now reliving as she looks at the blockers to her potential self. She gets out her phone and shows me a picture of Melly. It is definitely the same woman who popped into my head.

Weird.

I don't know what to think. The image of Melly inside my head was as clear to me as anything I have ever seen. It wasn't conjured by *my* brain; it's not an image in my memory. It definitely came into my mind from outside. So the logic is that it must have come from Rachel, on whom I had been concentrating intently. How that happened I have no idea. It goes against everything I think I know about communication, about how brains work, but I cannot doubt the veracity of my own experience. I categorically saw Melly. I am officially freaked out.

That is the power of Constellations; the process taps you into new ways of knowing, which are not rational, or conscious, or the way we usually know, but are no less real for that. Constellators call this 'tapping into the field'.

Being part of this Constellation (and many others since – I reckon it is about as much fun as you can have with your clothes on) enabled me to see that we are all connected, linked in ways we aren't usually aware of. That we can 'tap into the field' and use it to tune in to each other. Scientists now think that people may be able to sense each other in the way that flocks of birds communicate seemingly instantly when, for instance, murmurations change direction. Or whales locate each other and navigate over huge distances.

Many cultures throughout history have known the power of this connection; indeed, we all experience it sometimes when we think of someone and they ring us up, or they feel, like my heron, almost conjured by our thought; it is just in our super-rational world that we reject such possibilities. In fact, the cutting edge of physics now is all about how nothing exists in separation but only in relation to other particles or forces. Maybe what seems whacky – or becomes clear when taking psilocybin, when this connectedness is very evident – is actually true.

When it came to my own turn to be the subject in the constellation and I looked at my future self, I was overcome by sorrow. When I tried to feel my way into where I was and what was behind me, I also drew a blank. When I thought of my husband and children, that felt comforting, solid. But when I was told to think about my parents and birth family, there was only sadness and a vacuum. I intuited that that sadness, that emptiness, that hole, that void, was maybe something I needed to explore, process, shed. That it was holding me back.

It was the start of some profound and life-changing work. I had seven years of therapy in my twenties, so it is not as if I hadn't tried to deal with this void before. But the combination of the Constellations and the retreat made me delve into areas I had always feared to explore.

That week on retreat I used a lot of tissues. I wasn't the only one. Many of us there were in transition, or coping with something startlingly new, or stubbornly old, and sad. There is such friendship and connection to be found in our fellow travellers at such times.

During one exercise I apologised for being 'too much': at that time I felt 'too' everything – too noisy, too naughty, too big, too fat ... too me. In the circle afterwards a man who has since become my friend said, 'Never think you are too much, Eleanor. You are such a life force. Perfect as you are. It makes me sad to see you say sorry for something so special; that "muchness", that "exuberance", it is your gift. Don't apologise for it, ever again! Promise me!'

The whole group nodded in agreement as I wept copiously.

I resolved never to shrink myself again. Never to make myself small to make it easier for others. Never to feel that I should take up less space. Something women are particularly prone to! I decided instead to own what and how I am in the world, to revel in it. To feel happy about being 'stout', planted, resolutely and totally me – and to be proud of my stoutness. In fact, that 'stout' quality, feeling grounded, rocklike, solid, I now believe is a very important part of the Queenager journey: learning to accept and love ourselves just as we are, in our true essence, and to feel proud to take up that space, to be truly ourselves. Stout. Whole. It was a revelation.

Try it. Try just saying to yourself: 'I am enough, just as I am.' It's powerful.

That afternoon we went back to our rooms with the suggestion that we write a list of all the things we wanted to shed. The idea being that that evening we would symbolically burn the list, leave behind all those painful things, on a ceremonial fire.

I tearfully wrote a list of all those childhood feelings of not being enough, not feeling loved or wanted just for being me. With it I also wrote down all the things that the desperate need to feel seen and valued – validated by the world – had caused me to do. Some filled me with guilt. My numbness had certainly allowed me to behave in ways that had hurt others. Feeling into that, seeing it, repenting it, behaving differently as a result, has been a big part of my midlife shift. I realise how I had come to value achievement over nearly everything else, because growing up it was the only currency my family responded to. When I achieved was the only time that I ever felt seen, or valued. But that kind of external achievement will never fill the void; to come to terms with that we have to do the emotional work. And it hurts!

That evening at the ceremony, when it was my turn, I stepped forward, read out the list and threw the piece of paper on the fire. It felt good to watch all that pain, that old incarnation of myself, burn, vaporise in the flames. It felt good to witness it go, though even at the time I wasn't sure it could be that easy! (And it hasn't proved to be.) It wasn't the end of those feelings – not by a long shot. Those old patterns are hard to shift. But allowing ourselves to see them, writing them down, having the intention to behave in a new way, is definitely the beginning of the transformation.

Indeed, those few days on retreat at Broughton Hall were the start of a deeper unpeeling, a pruning. A sense of chopping back a hard shell, a carapace, a kind of armour which had masked a deeper me. Each trailing tendril that was chopped off hurt. Each past pain, the injury I had caused others, the numbness I had inflicted on myself – they could only be removed by being dissolved – in saline solution. In my tears.

It was the start of my cocoon time. Where I changed from being one iteration of myself to something new. What Clare Dubois – of the Sistering workshop – calls being 'putty'. In the chrysalis. In a kind of between state, neither one thing nor another. It was a start. I've said it before but I'll say it again: change is difficult. It means burrowing into places we'd rather avoid, excavating old wounds, sloughing off the scar tissue that has made us numb. But the weeks that I spent on retreat, digging deeper, trying to work out what I *really* felt, who I really was after all those years of being what everyone else wanted me to be, *were* the beginning of my rebirth, my becoming, the start of the hard work. The sore, teary, uncertain beginning of a whole new phase of my life. The necessary cocoon, the chrysalis period before the ongoing rebirth and growing of new wings.

During that week one of the other members of the circle was an American woman called Dianne. She had reached out to me with a wordless hug on one occasion when I wept, and held my hand. I just knew she understood, that she was carrying some deep pain of rejection too. One night at dinner we sat together – and she told me her story. Back then I had no idea that I was going to write this book. But her words went deep; her tale was so inspirational about midlife becoming, overcoming early rejection and metamorphosing at fifty, that I knew I wanted to share it somehow, even then. So here it is.

Dianne grew up in a strict Mormon community in Los Angeles. She was adopted and never knew her birth parents or anything about them. She became a mother herself very young, 'because I just wanted to be truly related to someone. When my first child was born I felt love for the first time in my life – this was someone who shared my blood. That instant soul connection was a huge thing for me.'

Dianne was born in a Salvation Army hospital and put up for adoption by LA County Foster Care. She was picked by a family by the time she was four months old. But having had four children herself, she knows the rupture that happened deep inside when she was separated from her mother. 'I carry sadnesses for which I have no words, which are pre-verbal.'

Dianne is a harpist and was part of a group that took music therapy into hospitals. Playing one day in the White Memorial Hospital in LA she realised it was the institution on her birth certificate and decided to try to trace her blood parents.

She met her birth mother for the first time on the day she turned fifty. 'I was disappointed I didn't feel a strong connection, or recognition.' It turned out that Dianne was one of four babies her mother had had adopted. 'But she did tell me the name of my birth father.' That he was a surfer, and they met at high school.

Dianne rang the high school and it turned out that the administrator knew her father. A few days later she rang back, saying she had found Dianne's dad, that he was homeless but his surfing buddies were going to bring him to a restaurant to meet her.

This meeting was different. 'I immediately felt an affinity with him. Just like I had with my first baby. I just felt: this is where I come from. He looked like me. He just felt like kin. My adoptive family had always been kind to me but they never felt like me, like my people. This man just immediately did. He took me in his arms and hugged me and said: "Oh, honey!" It felt like I had come home.'

Dianne says that it was as if the cassette which had been the first fifty years of her life 'suddenly unravelled out of my brain and could never be put back in again'. Everything changed in that instant. 'I started spending time with him, hanging out in the canyon in California where he lived, just lying together looking up at the stars. My father just lived in nature, in the flow of the waves; he felt connected to all things. He and his friends had tried to live in a new way, cultivating their own vegetables, being vegetarian, living in a commune outside the stream of American life.'

Dianne's husband was a Mormon bishop, she had been American 'Mother of the Year'. Until she met her father her life had been super-respectable, prescribed by duty, family, the temple. But when she met her father, everything shifted. She felt like she'd been given a 'get out of jail free' card. Her dad hadn't just been a surfer but one of the biggest drug dealers in the US, part of the Brotherhood of Eternal Love – the group of surfers and hippies who lived in the canyon and hung out with Timothy Leary – who created a pure form of LSD known as 'Orange

Sunshine' and smuggled marijuana in their surfboards. The Grateful Dead and Jimi Hendrix played at a festival in the canyon while 25,000 tabs of 'Orange Sunshine' were dropped on the crowd from a cargo plane. 'My father was in the middle of all that "Turn On, Tune In, Drop Out" counterculture,' Dianne says. He had been arrested sixty-five times, had no possessions because he just wanted to live in nature, surf and do his thing. It couldn't have been any more different from her life (she says she was the kind of mum who wound up the windows when they drove past tramps) but that all changed. 'My dad just felt like home,' she repeats.

For Dianne, meeting her dad marked a profound spiritual shift. Having been adopted by Mormons, she had grown up surrounded by religion. But her dad 'just oozed real spirituality, he just resonated with me. I had such a huge download from him without knowing it – he changed everything.'

Finding her father at fifty caused Dianne to completely change her life. 'I went to see a therapist, who said, "It's like you've been living in a thicket and you've finally come out and seen the moon. You can either go back in and put on your apron and pretend you haven't seen it, or you can make a change."'

Her father died within months of their meeting; he had already been ill when she found him. But she says he is with her all the time, that she feels his 'special energy, some imprint of the utopian society they were trying to build. A vision of a better world.' Meeting her father, she says, was the first time she understood what love was. 'I loved my children but I decided I had to leave my husband and my life. Yes, it was painful. I walked away from everything: all my friends, my life of fifty years, the place I'd grown up; we sold our house.'

It wasn't easy. Dianne says it was traumatic for her and for her grown children, but that they could immediately see how much happier she was. 'I got a whole clean slate. I started again and became a completely different person. I needed a different life. I spent fifty years as someone dutiful, who wasn't fully alive. And I just thought, I'm done. We need to show all the girls and the women coming after us that women can change anytime. They can just become something new. We need to model that for our daughters, that the journey is long and it can be different from what's prescribed for us.'

Like me, Dianne hadn't felt restless but numb, and she hadn't even realised what was missing. 'Too many women make those big life decisions – the husband, the career, the kids – when they are too young to know what they are choosing, before their brains are even formed. I ended up with a life that was so not me. We are the first generation of women to be healthy enough to choose something different at fifty.'

Secret: Sometimes we need to turn off our logical brain and follow our instincts, our heart – let it take us somewhere new. That could be into a different person from the one we thought we were. Play around with different ways of knowing, spend time in nature, push out of your normal comfort zone, face your fears and leave them behind. You just might emerge so much happier! I did.

The universe has our back

By this point my life was very different from how it had been. I started every day by meditating for thirty minutes and at noon, come rain or shine, I would go to the pond. I'd started to joke that I spent so much time every day on self-care – what with the meditating and the swimming and the Pilates twice a week – that I barely had time to do anything else. Interestingly, though, my productivity massively ramped up. I found I could write articles quicker because I was surer about what I wanted to say. There was less doubt and anxiety. I'd also noticed that good things began to come my way in terms of the business and the people in my life. The more I relaxed and went with the flow, the more I was calm and stout and truly myself, the more things seemed to come towards me rather than me trying to grab them. I'd begun to be glad that I had left my big job and set off on a new path. I was feeling my way towards a new version of myself.

But I would still sometimes find myself overcome with sadness. I would get frustrated that, despite all the work I'd been doing on shedding my childhood demons, they kept coming back. I would shed stuff on a retreat, or suchlike, and then find myself, annoyingly, right back in the overwhelmingly teary, sad place, like I was on a circular loop.

I was climbing down the steps at the pond on a wintry day when the water, trees and even sky seemed brown and grey, when I bumped into the woman who had taught me pregnancy yoga two decades ago. Ayala is a truly inspirational teacher; it was because of the way she had taught me to trust, surrender and breathe that I had had two natural births.

We swam together and she said she was leading a seven-day-long, completely silent retreat a few weeks hence. Gently, she said she thought I might find it helpful. I'd been telling her about my spiritual journey-ings; she had been in Peru taking ayahuasca on a similar kind of pilgrimage.

To be honest, I wasn't convinced by the idea of a week in silence. I am a chatterbox, I talk, I tell stories. The mere thought of being silent for so long filled me with terror. And I am no yogi; seven hours of yoga and meditation a day with no chat sounded intense, and I hadn't done any yoga seriously since those pregnancy sessions – and my eldest daughter was by then twenty!

And yet this whole journey has been about serendipity, saying yes to what the universe offers. Trusting that a door was being opened by that person in that moment for a reason. So I swallowed my trepidation about the silence and decided to go anyway.

The long, dark train ride to Totnes was punctuated by WhatsApps from my siblings, taking bets on how long I could last without speaking. No one thought I could be quiet (least of all me). It wasn't just not speaking to the fellow retreatants, either; it was 'suggested' that I hand in my phone for the entire time I was there. This wasn't a suggestion, really, it was kind of a command. The week ahead was to be a digital and communication silence too.

As luck would have it, the friend who had said I should 'never think I was too much' lived near the retreat centre. He collected me from the train and we went for a yomp by the Devon coast and ate treacle tart while he kindly convinced me that I could manage the silence that was to come. Oh, the joy of new friends, a new tribe who know a new version of you and what that person can do. Sometimes before we even know it ourselves!

He was right. Over the following days I surprised myself. I discovered that silence was indeed golden. That I like silent Eleanor; without all the noise and fuss, she's mellow and thoughtful. She notices the colours of the leaves, golden on the beeches, tawny on the oaks. She sits and watches the wind blow the clouds into different shapes and loves how the full moon throws shadows on the river and the hills.

On the retreat, we began every morning at 6.45 with a silent meditative walk to the River Dart to plunge into the fast-flowing waters. On the morning after the full moon I swam far out to see its pearly-orb double, simultaneously in the water around me and high in the sky. A huge seal joined me in the river, his whiskery face human in scale. As he loomed near, one of the other women yelped with fear. But to me he felt benign. It was a moment of deep wonder and blessing to be in the water with a creature wild and free, and as big as me.

But in a stark reminder that light and dark, Yin and Yang, always exist together, my exultant joy at swimming with the seal and the moons flipped suddenly into near panic. As I turned to head back to the jetty I felt the current tugging, strong, inexorable, against me – the tidal River Dart flowing to the sea. I began to swim hard, head down, swift strokes, towards the jetty and safety. A pulse of fear ripped through my mind and body – would I be too cold to make it? The water was chilly, and I had already been in longer than I'd intended or was sensible given the temperature because the moon was so beautiful.

I looked to the bank; the oak tree opposite stayed stubbornly level even as I swam faster. I was getting nowhere. Heart pounding. Maximum effort. Still no progress.

Then I changed tack, swimming across the current away from the bank to get out of the strongest flow. Slowly, slowly, I began to make headway.

Sometimes to go forwards, we must go sideways. And sometimes we just have to trust, keep trying, keep going, even when the tide against us seems insurmountable. I was grateful to the woman beside me also swimming hard. In silence. Her encouraging smile. The comfort of being in it together.

I was very grateful to make it back.

I learnt to eat in silence. Food tastes better with no distractions. I would think about the journey each bit of food had been on. Where the chickpea had been grown, the cow who had made the milk, the tree where someone had plucked the apple. The journey and effort involved in getting all of this goodness onto my plate. It was restful being surrounded by friendly women who couldn't speak. I learnt who I liked; some smiled or caught my eye, in shared humour or under-standing. Sometimes we cried and comforted each other, wordlessly with a squeezed hand, a smile, a stolen hug.

The liberation from small talk was great. We unhooked from our normal stories. Without the 'Where do you live? What do you do? Do you have kids?' cacophony of normal interaction, a deeper interplay began. Together we huffed and puffed and downward-dogged, through seven hours of yoga and meditation a day. That sounds like a lot but it felt eminently doable. Two three-hour yoga sessions (Iyengar in the morning, Yin in the afternoon) plus a pre-breakfast and after-dinner thirty-minute meditation. In the afternoon I would lie in my bed and feel where in my body emotions lurked and follow the stories that unfurled. That week was a deep dive into our inner selves, unpeeling the layers. Feeling into where in our bodies we hold the pain we'd usually rather not visit. Unearthing the wounds and sitting with them, quietly, with love, allowed me to peer deeper, understand more.

So what did I learn? Mainly self-compassion. I realised that often in my life I'll turn to my partner or my children and ask, and mean it: 'How do you feel, my love? What do you need, my love? How are you, really?' But until that week I don't think I'd ever lovingly asked that question of myself. I realised I'd been a hard taskmaster to myself. A tyrant, even – expecting long hours, ignoring my body, my tiredness, my intuition, even overriding, for decades, a deep sense of wrongness at what I was doing. I'd been living in a state of self-abnegation in order to appease the achievement god, driving myself on. I worked in a tough world, of machismo and extremes, sharp tongues and competition – with the benefit of hindsight I'm sure I was tough on others too.

Maybe I didn't ever ask how I really was back then because the answers would have been too dangerous. Because I wasn't ready to hear them. Because I was too driven. Trying too desperately to fill a huge hole inside me – what I could now see as a mega sense of lack – with ever more professional achievement. Using busyness and external success to mask the scary void inside me.

Now I am amazed that I lived at such odds with my deeper self for so long. I talk at Noon, and in many of the keynotes and speeches I do about Queenagers, about how we become the women we always wanted to be at fifty. On retreat I realised that that deeper becoming starts with truly asking ourselves what *we* want, what makes *us* happy (not everyone else we've been trying to please). And being brave (and feeling held and safe) enough to listen to the (often uncomfortable) answers. To see what we have been hiding from ourselves.

That week I dived deep into my body. The yoga provided a pathway to an inner listening, an awareness of where the tension is inside, where the sadness is held in the body. Some of you may have read *The Body Keeps the Score* – well, it's true. We don't have to have gone through PTSD levels of trauma for our bodies to keep track of our inner wounds.

I handed in my phone on the first night. Did not speak to anyone. Had no e-mails, or phone calls, or mindless scrolling for a week. All normal distractions were stripped back. Even books or the radio were removed. And what was given the space to emerge through the physical practice and the quiet were all the bits of me I usually try not to think about; the bits which are painful, the darkness we usually run from.

The teacher, Ayala, urged us just to sit with what was there, with love. To go towards it. To sit beside it. To soften around it. Most of all to allow ourselves to feel it and let the tears flow. One woman said later that she'd found the feeling of tears running down her face into her chin to be like a caress, that after months of bottling up her grief for her dead mother it felt liberating to let it go. That the tears felt peaceful. Comforting.

I located old wounds in my body. Spent time feeling them, unpeeling the layers of them, going towards the suffering and sitting quietly with it with love. I found that, by allowing all of it in, there was healing and revelation.

That's not to say it wasn't dark. It was. At one point I broke down; sobbed uncontrollably in the middle of the class. I had a profound sense of not being able to comfort myself, of not being able to cope, of this feeling of abandonment, of hopelessness, being bigger and sadder than I could manage on my own. Of being overwhelmed and hopeless. At a loss. I sat cross-legged on my mat, shaking with sobs and sorrow. Ayala came and wrapped her arms around me and hugged me, pulling me to her breast and crooning over me. 'It's okay, my love,' she said again and again, until it passed.

Revisiting the memory, the tears still flow. It went very deep. Pre-words. I asked my mother about it later and she recounted how, when I was nine months old, she and my dad left me for two or three weeks in London with a new nanny I didn't know while they went to America for a wedding. She said that when they left, I was smiley and could sit up. But that when they came back, I had regressed and just lay in my cot helplessly.

I have always felt somewhere inside me a deep sadness; it would ambush me, often around the time of my period, leaving me weeping and raw – anathema to my normal bouncy self. I had always attributed it to the pain of my parents divorcing when I was five, but I learnt during that morning that the deep wound, that profound sense of abandonment, of hopelessness, had come way earlier. I located its source, that feeling of not being able to comfort myself, that nobody was coming, that I was alone and untended. Helpless. I felt in some way that it had finally, at fifty, been tended, healed at least to some extent – by Ayala.

Some wounds are unfixable; we don't get over them but they become part of our warp and weft like knots in the trunk of a tree. By locating the source of mine and understanding it, it has become easier. Not gone. It can still ambush me. But I don't fear it annihilating me anymore.

At lunch that day at the retreat one of the other women passed me a note: 'Thank you for crying for all of us,' it said. I cried for them, but I also cried for me.

The beauty of this experience was that I felt no shame in my distress, only comfort and support. For years I had sought to hide, to camouflage, to surround with armour and achievement that deep weakness. But that week I found there was strength in that total vulnerability, that openness to everything, to embracing complexity and all the different strains of who we are – that there is light in the darkness. Maybe, in fact, as the Yin-Yang sign suggests, the light in the middle of the darkness, the love and support that we find there, shines the brightest of all.

At the opening of the retreat Ayala read these words of Mary Haskell's to the author of that wonderful book, *The Prophet*, Kahlil Gibran: 'Nothing you become will disappoint me; I have no preconception that I'd like to see you be or do. I have no desire to foresee you, only to discover you. You cannot disappoint me.' So many of us have been programmed to please, to be what others want us to be; I loved that injunction just to be ourselves, however that manifested. That all was welcome, everything was okay. That nothing we did, or were, could disappoint.

For me the midlife journey has been one of trusting that, even when downswings come, the universe has our back. My learning is to lean into the uncertainty, welcome in the unknown, embrace the flow. To try to live as I do when I float on the water, trusting it's got me; that I am held between pond and sky. This lesson is hard-won. It's easy to slip into despair, to tears, to anxiety, but now when I face a setback I try to take a pause, a breath, a beat. To reach for love and kindness to myself. I have felt on a cellular level that what feels like the darkest blow can with time be the right thing, the light thing. That disappointment and pain in the moment don't necessarily mean all is lost – indeed, in the greater weave it might just be for the best.

Secret: In the darkest moments shines the brightest light. Allowing ourselves to be truly seen and comforted, to go towards the hurt rather than run away from it, is where the healing lies. The pain is the portal.

PART SEVEN

BECOMING

The black wings of the cormorant skim so close that the breeze ruffles my hair. It dives and disappears. I count slowly, scanning the oil-glossy water, noticing the green tints in the black surface, wondering where in this wide watery expanse it has gone. Is it even now beneath me, its long dinosaur beak lurking in the dark depths below my stomach? Can it see in the murkiness below to catch its prey? Where will it resurface? When?

I dive down; there is an exquisite thrill from the water's chill on my head. I point my toes to the sky, knowing the weight of my legs will force me deeper down. It is gloomy here in the depths, brown and cloudy – even with my eyes open I am swimming blind. As I head for the surface sight returns, the colours turn from muddy brown to yellow, then green and suddenly the white-grey of sky. Near the surface the water is deceptively clear. As I glide back up, I feel I too can swoosh and fly in the water, gravity be damned. I am like a bird, weightless, exultant, free.

But not for long. My maximum immersion is a count of five or ten; after that I must return to the air. The cormorants dive for over fifty. I love the way they vanish then pop up far away. Endless sport to watch the trepidation on the faces of other swimmers. Where did it go? When will it return? Will it? On other days the cormorants perch on the orange plastic buoys, their pterodactyl looks a jarring contrast; ancient and modern. They dry their huge jet-black wings in the autumn sun. They don't have waterproof feathers like ducks, they need to sunbathe to dry. Like us they are semi-aliens, guests, in this watery world.

It feels right that, mythologically, cormorants are symbols of unease, of uncertainty. That three together are a warning; of greed, of deception – of the deep lies we tell ourselves. They are beautiful but also sinister, crow-like. They speak of ancient times, of dinosaurs destroyed, of the dives we take into the depths and the currents that linger there. Tides that run deep, unconscious motivations, those parts we hide from ourselves, which can emerge from the depths to rock us, knock us off balance. When we least expect it. When we think they've gone. Those deep wounds which don't seem to heal however much work we do. However hard we try.

So cormorants are now synonymous for me with what lies beneath. The underlying programming, the deep currents of conditioning in which we have swum, which have shaped us as women, often without us realising. Without us ever consciously knowing. You see, we women have been groomed by patriarchy; melded into the shape that most suits those who have ruled the world for the last two thousand years. We've been physically weaker, emotionally more turbulent, but we wield power over procreation and family; so we have been controlled. Made the legal possessions of men through marriage, trained from childhood to be helpmeets, pleasers. These same dark forces removed the stories of wise old women, of healers, of midwives, from our cultural narratives. Replaced them instead with tales of witches and fearful hags, wicked stepmothers, Cruella de Vil.

The most important thing to remember is that this isn't our fault; it's a product of the world we were raised in. One of the great female icons of our generation's childhood – for good or ill – the woman who took up more newspaper front pages and general oxygen than anyone else, was Diana, Princess of Wales. Our parents' generation talk about where they were when Kennedy was shot; a similar moment for us was the death of Diana following a car crash in the Pont de l'Alma tunnel in Paris in 1997. As an editor I covered many huge events – 9/11, elections, wars – but Diana's death stands out. The reaction to her death was extraordinary; people loved her, felt they knew her, saw their own lives and struggles reflected in her. She had been held up as a symbol of femininity to the whole country. That was why hordes of people mobbed the streets when she died, why her last journey from Westminster Abbey to the island where she is buried was attended by millions lining the route.

If she were still alive, Diana would be a Queenager. When she got engaged in 1981, she was nineteen, a child, a lamb to the slaughter, all girlish charm, huge eyes and flirty glances at the paparazzi. When she got engaged to Charles, she was asked what her hopes for the future were: 'I just want to be a good wife and mother,' she said.

I was ten then. Princess Di was the most famous woman in the world; her aspirations were shared by many women whose identity was still grounded in their role as carers, supports to men and their offspring. Diana was held up to us as the *ne plus ultra* of a female archetype – everything we were told we wanted to be. She was all over the news, splashed across magazines – a generation of women imagined arriving at their weddings in enormous over-the-top meringue frocks and veils, riding in a glass coach just like Diana (and that other retro princess sidekick, Cinderella). That seems shockingly old-fashioned to me now; like my granny talking about taking a horse-drawn gig to church. I would never talk in that way about a woman's role to my own daughters.

But those old attitudes about what a woman should be were drummed into our Queenager generation. Just take that global phenomenon, the Brownies. I had a look through a Brownie guidebook from my childhood. It is all about women being good hostesses, ironing shirts and making meals as selflessly and quietly as possible. It is patriarchal propaganda – women as silent helpmeets, being trained never to expect praise or to think of themselves but just to shut up and get on with serving others. There are badges in how to bake scones, make salads (they are big on salads and exercises – Brownies need to be attractive and definitely not fat for their husbands). The most points were awarded for being a good hostess and generally looking after everyone else and putting one's own needs last. This isn't from the 1950s; it was published towards the end of the 1970s, when Queenagers like us were growing up. I bet Diana was a Brownie.

These tropes – putting others' needs ahead of our own, not asking for recognition, being helpmeets – were bred into us. Margaret Thatcher might have been prime minister, but we Queenagers were still raised not to put ourselves forwards, to serve humbly and do our best quietly. To ask for no reward. No wonder so many Queenagers still feel out of their comfort zone when they are asked to speak up or put themselves forwards in the workplace. No wonder so many Queenagers feel pulled in all directions. One woman described the inside of her mind as being like a computer with fifty tabs open as she juggled work, family, her mum's Alzheimer's. No wonder so many Queenagers put their own needs and desires last. Or forget that they even have them!

That early conditioning, the need to have a badge to prove you could do something, that whole ethos of there being a 'right' way to do things and women being judged for doing it wrong is so destructive. Destructive both to notions of agency, and self; it turbocharges our inner critic. That scolding inner voice is something I see so often in women in my circles. Scratch the surface and so many of us have a huge sense of lack, of not being enough, of not doing it right, that we should try harder, do more, be more.

It's why we find it hard to do what *we* want; become the women *we* want to be. That conditioning holds us back. If we are to shed these internal earworms in midlife we need to understand where they come from. Be kinder and gentler to ourselves. Dare to ask ourselves what *we* like, what *we* want. One woman put it to me like this: 'All I've done is work and do the kids and look after my elderly mum for as long as I can remember. I don't *know* what I like anymore.' Another woman told me she felt like she was 'sleepwalking through my life, that I haven't chosen any of it'. She said it was so long since she'd done anything for herself – rather than for her kids, boss or partner – that she'd practically forgotten what she used to like and desire and want. Another, whose children have both left home and who is single, described walking round the supermarket: 'I've bought what everybody else wants and likes – blueberries for my daughter, coleslaw for the little one – for so long that I've forgotten what I like, what I want!'

Enough of that. It's time to put ourselves centre stage.

The feminist revolution is only a part of the way through. We are told a constant lie that we have equality, that everything is fixed; I was first told that when I went to university. It was rubbish. They might have (on sufferance) let women into my Oxford college in 1989, but I was never taught by a female tutor, and there weren't any pictures of women on the wall. It was an entirely male zone, where women had been grudgingly admitted. They gave us the lanyard but that didn't mean we had equality. Just because we were allowed in – finally – didn't mean it was set up for us. We didn't have equality then. And we don't now. We've had the vote for one hundred years, but only three female prime ministers in the UK and no female presidents in the US. Laws don't make it so: we've had the Equal Pay Act since the 1970s but women are still paid less than men for the same job. And as we are seeing with Roe v Wade, even the legal protections women have over our own bodies, won with such struggle, can be revoked, wound back. The fight for equality is ongoing.

Understanding these forces, getting to grips with the currents that have shaped us, is crucial if we are going to move into our power, into our prime, in midlife. We women are like lobsters who are being slowly boiled in a pot. We don't even realise the temperature is rising, that we are living in dangerously hot water, which is turning us pink, distorting our essences, because we were born into it.

That is why we need to understand the bigger currents at play, to become conscious of what is being done to us. As Simone de Beauvoir said in her ground-breaking book *The Second Sex*: 'One is not born, but rather becomes, a woman.' By that she means that we are conditioned, shapeshifted into roles that serve patriarchy. Think of it as a kind of slow process of psychological foot-binding; where we women are taught from birth to make ourselves smaller, quieter, thinner, prettier, more *pleasing* because men prefer it – and it's easier for them – if we are that way.

We women must extract ourselves from the metaphorical lobster pot before it is too late. Before we are cooked! Many of us don't realise quite how cooked we've been until we become Queenagers. It is only when the limited cards we are given by patriarchy, the power that comes with being fertile and fuckable, wanes that we realise that women's rainbow of qualities, our intelligence, our competence, our kindness, our knowledge, our intuition, are of no interest to the male lens of our society once the two qualities that interest men have gone. It is why older women have so little clout or visibility in our society. This was summed up for me by a Queenager in one of our Noon Circles: 'I've traded on being beautiful, being a mother, since my twenties. I've had two husbands, have five children, but now they have all left home and I feel I have no role. I feel beached. Like, what do I do now?' Understanding this, unpicking it and valuing women for *all* that they are, not just what men have wanted us to be, is crucial.

Queenager-hood is all about moving beyond patriarchal expect-ations and definitions of a woman's worth into a new way of valuing ourselves. Of moving into *our* purpose – finding work or a cause that fulfils and motivates us. Embracing our creativity, not just to bring forth life but ideas, businesses, books, charities, art. Of becoming new kinds of role models of what women can be to our younger sisters. Most of all, at this age we become wiser, we move into wisdom, by understanding the way we have been shaped, moulded, created by our society. By seeing the forces that act on us we can move beyond them, reach for and find our own power by founding our own organisations, or doing work that is meaningful, or going back to the dreams we had when we were younger which were derailed by life and looking after others.

Several childfree women in this book talk about establishing different narratives around what is valuable in a woman: creativity, nurturing future generations through mentoring, exploring our passions. Once we are beyond fifty and invisible to the male gaze and the male lens through which we have seen ourselves, it is as if we are all childfree. After all, even if we have had kids, they are gone and grown up, living their own lives, making their own mistakes. This gives all Queenagers a chance for self-actualisation, to become the women we always wanted to be; to embrace ourselves in our fullness. In our stoutness, our wholeness. Becoming all that we are and can be. This has not yet been modelled in our society, partly because there have not been women in midlife like us with the lifespan and resources to move into a new chapter at fifty-plus. But we are here now and we are creating new maps, new signposts, a new landscape of possibilities for what we can be at this point in our lives and beyond, for the women who come after us. We need to model the joys of Queenager-dom for our daughters, so that they look forward to it rather than dreading it. This matters.

A meditation teacher once said to me: 'You cannot fly like an angel, journey into spiritual realms, into your power and your wisdom, if your arms, your wings, are wrapped around others.' I love that. So many of us women have spent the last three decades caring for others, wrapping our wings around them. Now is the time when we can stop using our arms in the service of others and instead use our wings, our longevity, our consciousness of our power and possibility, to soar, to fly, to inspire others to follow, to become. That is the very essence of this book.

New beginnings

Hundreds of women are queuing for the pond, grouching about the hour-long wait. Days like these annoy me. They shouldn't. I know I should welcome the excitable girls and fair-weather swimmers who flock here when the temperature rises. Feel happy that they are venturing into my watery Eden. I don't, though. I feel invaded. There are no concessions given to those of us who swim every day – who love the pond even when it's raining and 4 degrees on a dank February afternoon. It feels unfair that our unwavering loyalty counts for nothing. That on sunny days we stand in – endless – line with everyone else. Yet even while I wait here feeling a bit grumpy, I am aware that above me the birds are singing. That it is good for me to cultivate patience, to stand in line. If I'm honest, it's still a bit of a novelty to embody this new version of me. An hour-long queue would have been unconscionable to my old self.

I used to boast about being 'the most impatient woman in the world'. I travelled through my days so fast, gobbling up so much interaction – electronic and physical – that any delay felt like an insult. If I had to wait, I used to want to yell: 'Do you not know how busy I am? How much I cram into every possible moment? How valuable my time is?' I was like a tired toddler screaming for attention. Mainlining entitlement. There was status in extreme busyness; in my time being so in demand, so precious. For decades that achievement masked the massive existential hole inside me. If I just kept on running at full tilt,

I was too busy to feel sad – or to feel anything, really. Except hectic, needed, important, numb. It's a powerful, addictive drug, busyness and power. One that doesn't come with a health warning – but should!

It has taken three years to stop being that person, to learn to slow down. To notice the way the light refracts off ripples in the water, creating a disco-strobe effect on the lower branches of the trees. Or to catch the iridescent azure of the kingfisher as he flashes past. I have learnt, through daily immersion in this place, of the possibility of these moments. Familiarity has bred a hyper-alertness to what might appear, an attunement to subtle changes, to beauty. I find myself pointing out these treasures to others, initiating them into the pond wonders.

In our normal lives we 'glove' ourselves. Hide our true natures. Maybe we don't say exactly what we really feel, or we ram our round selves into square holes. Or we screen who we really are, what we actually think or truly want, out of a sense of lack or unworthiness, or fear of rejection. Or we just numb ourselves with stimulation and distraction so we can forget what we truly feel, or even who we really are. Squishing ourselves into the shape the world requested. After a while we are so gloved, so numb, so contorted, we lose sight of our real selves. Of what we could be.

I feel like I have become 'ungloved', as the poet Mark Nepo puts it. That I have sloughed off the callouses, the barriers, the armour that used to insulate me from the world. That pruning has been a deeply painful process. There have been times – particularly while on silent retreat, with all distractions removed, where I have had to spend days on end just with myself – when the regret and hurt have overwhelmed me. Where I have been incapacitated by sorrow as I confronted my trespasses and been comforted by compassionate strangers just as I have also tended to them. But the corollary of that, the upside of having delved and sat in the darkness and wept, is a new incredible sensitivity to the world. Its bliss and its agony. A sense of opening up, feeling everything. Letting it all in. I suppose it is like the difference between immersion in the cold water in a neoprene wetsuit and the prickling intensity of the chill on bare skin.

This journey for me has been all about 'ungloving' – relearning how to feel, connect, reflect. Discovering how to be at ease, comfortable and safe within my own skin but also with those around me. To be reborn into the world with a sense of internal spaciousness; a sense of having come home within my own mind. Enough just as I am; safe and whole at last.

But the journey isn't just one of personal contentment. Now that I am more open, aligned, truthful and purposeful, I find I am braver. That I can have a bigger, more benign effect on the world.

I've learnt that the way we do anything is the way we do everything. That it all matters. That we can't just park the bits of ourselves that we don't like, or are hurt, or behave badly, somewhere else. Because there is nowhere else. Or other. No 'us and them'. We are all linked. All the same. Part of one hyper-connected planet in which we all play our own part. By fixing ourselves we show up differently. We can receive love, give love – be love in the world – and begin to inspire others to do the same. We can start to be the change we want to see. To hold the hope that we can all do better.

All of that is here, at the pond. The community of women. The easy smiles. The friendship. The true sense of being stripped back, naked, open. To the good stuff and the sadness too.

To get into the water is to enter the singularity, the shared space, with all the women who have been here before. It reminds me of the huge fortune of being here now in this life, on this planet, watching the wondrous heron soar over the water, wings outstretched, its wing touching my cheek.

The pond strips me bare. Cleansing not just body but mind. It is freedom. In the water all shapes are possible.

As I walk home, up the muddy path, under the horse chestnut trees, the world is spangly again, my very blood sparkles. I hear the parakeets screech, chivvying each other from tree to tree. I sing and whistle with elation; my post-swim smile so broad, strangers grin back at me.

Pond-joy is contagious.

Secret: How could you dismantle your armour and open your true self to the world? What could that look like? What would you be if you were no longer afraid?

Much more to come

It is Christmas and I am sitting with the same friend who was there for me after my fall. This time it is not warm but wintry; we are not drinking tepid Pimm's, but hot tea from a thermos, on a bench by the pond. Another bench, the same friend. This time it is snowy.

We have just swum together in the icy water. It was so cold we both felt scared of venturing in, even with boots, gloves and woolly hats. Yet, determined, we slithered to the edge and navigated the frosty steps, ropes frozen solid, icicles dangling. Steam rose from our warm bodies. Ducks skidded drunkenly on the ice – there was only a small swimming hole today, carved out of the frozen expanse. The cold burns as we venture in. Today it isn't about swimming any distance but just the immersion. Doing it at all. We swim from one set of steps to the other – and back. Daring ourselves to go again. Giggling with the insanity of it. Shouting out warnings not to cut ourselves on the jagged ice. Feeling the cold which burns so it almost feels hot.

We emerge at last and clamber out onto the deck, which is slithery and covered with grit and salt. We hug each other tight. Triumphant. Alive! We throw on layers of thermals and jumpers. Shiver into our coats and sit companionably on the bench, swigging tea and eating mince pies, home-made that morning. The sun is shining. The pond is shimmering. Above us each leaf and branch sparkles, frost-lit. We are exultant. Ecstatic. Way higher than happy. Our sobbing summer tryst in lockdown only two and a half years before feels a lifetime away.

We talk about that day. How lost I was, how sad, and about how far we have come. I thank her for being there for me, tell her how much she helped. We talk of the tribe of Queenagers who have supported me through it, Claire, the angel who invested in me and the business, and how her belief when I had none myself was a game-changer. We talk about how different we are, how reinvention really is possible. How even at fifty, or later, we can find a better self, an awakened self, a new life built out of the rubble of the old. That it takes courage, love, support, a new tribe and an openness to thinking differently, to trying new things – that shedding the old stuff hurts; particularly realising our trespasses and transgressions. But that with work it really is possible to feel truly that it is okay to be you, exactly as you are – right now.

It is hard. But possible.

Most of all, we talk about our friendship. All the times we have picked each other up, egged each other on, helped each other out – whether over kids, or work, or love. For over twenty-five years. And now here we are, Queenagers – with much more to come.

GLOSSARY

In writing this book and thinking about midlife I realised that we were missing a whole vocabulary which could describe and make concrete and accessible all the changes that happen and are possible at this time. I coined the term Queenager because I thought we needed a more optimistic and positive rebrand, but over the last few years I have also co-opted and created a whole new lexicon to describe some of the important aspects of midlife transformation. I provide this glossary here as a kind of index to many of the key concepts I have found helpful or illuminating, or that I have used in this book. I hope they will become the basis of a whole new cultural conversation about what a woman can be at this point and beyond, and give everyone a whole new way of thinking about the later stages of a woman's life. Enjoy!

4-Quarter Lives: Thought-leader Avivah Wittenberg-Cox talks about how, in the 100-year life which many of us will be lucky enough to live, the first quarter, Q1, is zero to twenty-four, getting educated, getting started; Q2 (25–49), the 'Age of Achievement', is where we tick off all the things we've been told we are supposed to be and want; Q3 (50–74) is the 'Age of Becoming' (*see below*) and Q4 (75–100), the winding down to the end.

***100-Year Life, The*:** Brilliant book by two London Business School professors, Lynda Gratton and Andrew Scott – says that we are all likely now to live to our century, but that we haven't worked out what that means in terms of how we structure or think about all that extra time, which, along with climate change, is one of the big challenges we all face. The old model of get educated, get a job, retire is no longer fit for purpose, but we haven't come up with a new framework to replace it with (*see* 4-Quarter Lives).

Age of Becoming: Fifty is when we become the women we always wanted to be. Carl Jung is reported to have once said: 'Life really does begin at forty. Up until then, you are just doing research.' Fifty is when we throw off the shackles of the programming, the 'shoulds' and 'society expects' and 'my parents wanted' and actually work out what it is we want to *be* before it is too late. Exciting, huh?

Burnout: When you have totally lost yourself, exhausted all your resources and need to stop (*see also* Fallowing, Less-ing and Wallowing).

Empty nest: When the kids go off to uni, or leave home completely. Feels a bit like stopping breast-feeding or when you leave your toddler at nursery for the first time, or they go to big school. Agony. Accompanied by often unwanted crying (particularly when you drop said child at their uni room for the first time) – you might have to wear sunglasses or disappear a lot to 'have a pee' (cry in the loo). Your child will think you are a total embarrassment. Don't worry, your feelings are entirely normal.

Fallowing: Intentionally taking time out to rest, recuperate and regenerate. This can be as simple as mooching about the house watching all those box sets you never had time for, fixing things that need it and generally taking time to do everything that has passed you by. But it could also be going on a retreat, or a walking holiday, giving yourself bigger time and space. This is not time-wasting, or goofing off, it is crucial to rejuvenation and transition. Inanna, the Assyrian goddess in the oldest of human myths, went down to the underworld and was hung on a hook, like a piece of meat in the dark. She regenerated – and came back queen of the world above and the world below. Sometimes we need to retreat into a metaphorical cave and sit in the silence and darkness and renew. Fallow times, like a field regaining its fertility through rest.

Forged in fire: Noon research shows that those Queenagers who have been through and survived the most are ultimately happiest. The wisdom in the room is the accumulation of all that life experience and knowledge – we will survive, and thrive.

Forty-niners: When testosterone levels for many women spike just before the menopause; a peak time for affairs ...

Gathering: Increasingly the task of a modern matriarch is to bring the disparate clan together. With so many of us living far away from family members, if cousins are to know each other and family to have some glue, they need to be brought together. How to do this and have so many different generations and personalities in the same place is often fraught, but necessary!

Gendered ageism: Where sexism meets ageism, particularly shit for women: that feeling that you have become invisible; when suddenly you are turning fifty and you get made redundant; the way older women disappear from all advertising and TV (unless they look freakishly young).

Glide to retirement: You get made a partner at fifty-five – but your firm insists you retire by sixty. So for one year you work five days a week, then the next four days a week, the next three and so on. Even if you actually feel you are just getting started, that after years of looking after everyone else you are in your prime and loving your job … hmmmm.

Happiness U-curve: According to research by economist David Blanchflower, unhappiness peaks at forty-seven in all cultures across the globe and then we feel better again as we age.

Healthspan: Like lifespan, but how long you stay healthy and able to move around and do all the things you want to do. To increase yours, try taking up some exercise, spending more time outside, eating fifteen different fruits and vegetables a week and including some of the Ks (kombucha, kimchi – fermented tea and cabbage respectively).

Hole, the: Success will never fill it up, or money, or external achievement. You have to work on the hole in your soul. You. No one can do it for you.

Joy: What brings you joy? What do you love doing, what makes you feel purposeful and content? Do more of it, prioritise it, use it as the stepping stones to your new life. It is a key tool of transition, a way of keeping you filled up, happy and on the right path. When it comes to this, the mantra is: 'Say yes to joy!' It is the way, the truth, your life.

Less-ing: Intentionally cutting back, doing less. Giving yourself more time.

Midlife maelstrom/midlife clusterfuck/midlife collision: When all problems hit at once – a tsunami of woes that assaults us between forty-five and fifty-five. Half of all Queenagers have experienced

at least five big life events, including: divorce, bereavement of
a partner, redundancy, bankruptcy, mental health issues, physical
health challenges, elderly parents (caring for/them dying), teenagers
(anxiety, self-harming, eating disorders, failure to launch), empty
nest, menopause. Sometimes these come in a paralysing cluster,
sending life off on a whole new tangent.

Nature: Being in nature suddenly becomes much more important at
this point. We start noticing the verdant hit of newly green leaves,
frothing blossom, ducks and ducklings, the beauty of sun sparkling
on water, wildflowers, herons, kingfishers, deer … It's as if we sud-
denly wake up to the wonder of the natural world, of Gaia and all our
wonderful planet gives us. It is a feeling of connection to the planet
that sustains us and to the interrelatedness of all things. That nature
isn't 'other', it is us, and finally we see it clearly and give thanks to it.

New tribe/new crew: If you want to become a new person then you
will find resistance from those around you who like you/need you/
expect you to remain in the same box you have always been in. To
make a shift, become the woman you always wanted to be, you
are going to need some new friends who know you in your new
incarnation – to find a new tribe. It's what we are creating at Noon!

Parental expectations: Sloughing them off at this point. Who are you
doing all of this for??

Personal sustainability: Tending to our personal sustainability is
essential because we can't go on harvesting ourselves forever (*see*
Burnout). If we've been doing a big job and/or raising a family/caring
for oldies or tricky teens, or basically running ourselves ragged for
whatever reason, at some point the tank runs dry. This is when
we need to engage in some personal rejuvenation (*see* Fallowing

and Wallowing). In order to regenerate we must go down into the dark. Sit and wait for the magic to happen, for us to replenish. Like resting land after ploughing and harvesting it for many seasons. Transitioning from one period of life to another requires some time out. Some deep rest and recuperation. This usually comes with some pain and sadness and shedding. That is okay. Feel your feelings. This too will pass. Just as the fields look muddy and barren and depleted in winter but spring back to life, so will you.

Pinch points: Yup, midlife certainly has some of these: divorce, bereavement, redundancy, elderly parents falling ill or needing new levels of support, tricky teens, your own health issues, menopause. And sometimes they all pile on at once (*see* Midlife maelstrom/ clusterfuck/collision) – but the good news is that once you get through the pinch points, it all gets better.

Prime: Welcome to your Queenager years, you are in your prime – reaping the rewards of all your hard work to date. As Oscar-winner Michelle Yeoh said: 'Ladies, don't let anyone tell you you are past your prime.' Enjoy yourself. This is where it gets good, ladies.

Pruning: Think about midlife as a reset. As if the universe is taking some big shears and lopping off all the long, trailing growth that is sapping your energy and no longer serves you. You are getting a good prune. It is painful having bits lopped off; particularly ones that you held dear. So grieve them, feel the agony – and let them go. You will spring back like a rose or a wisteria, stronger, pared back to your essence, raring to go with a strong green shoot of new life and regeneration.

Putty: When we stop being one version of ourselves and embark on a transformation, we enter a transition phase. We become putty, or stem cells; we are in the process of making ourselves into something new. Enjoy being fluid and finding your new mould. Try lots of things out, be open to everything. Don't hurry. You are putty. That is okay!

Queenager: In one of our Noon focus groups one of our midlife ladies described life in her fifties as, 'Feeling like a teenager, but in my own house, with good sheets and proper tea.' I spend quite a lot of time in Jamaica where they refer to older women as 'queens', so – with the benefit of thirty years of writing headlines – up popped 'Queenager'. It's a rebrand of women in midlife: this time can be whatever you want it to be.

Renegotiating your relationship: Therapists report that couples who stay together beyond midlife have a period of intense renegotiation: you want to paint and spend several months apart; he is addicted to middle-aged-man-in-Lycra cycling … you come to a deal that works for you both (or you don't).

Reskilling: Often, the more senior we become, the more people we have to do stuff for us. I ended up feeling like a giant baby. My cars would be booked, tickets provided, my social feeds were done by someone else – I never did anything for myself. When I started my own company and had to do my first Insta-Live I cried because I had no idea what to do. To stay engaged with the modern world, get yourself some digital smarts. These days I can StreamYard to my LinkedIn Live, run a community on Substack and even edit and resize my photos and create a post in WordPress. It's not that difficult and will make you feel back in charge of your next chapter.

The Revolt: That feeling we Queenagers get when we've simply had enough; enough of being pleasing, enough of being what everyone else wants us to be. When we say: 'No, stop, this is *my* time. I might not have that much time left, so I am going to start living for myself.' We pick up new passions, we get purposeful. We start becoming the women we were always supposed to be. (Thank you, Lucy Ryan, for the wisdom in your book *Revolting Women*, and your friendship.)

Shapeshifting: Women in particular get moulded into the shapes that fit everyone around us. At midlife the shape we have occupied can feel 'cabined, cribbed, confined', as Shakespeare put it. Our midlife journey is to find our true shape, the life we would be living if *we* chose it rather than being put in a box that suits everyone else. Remember, when you try to shapeshift, the system around you will endeavour to push you back into your old shape – it suits them. Expect resistance. Push on with your shapeshifting. We've got you! You've got this!

Silver splitters: The trend for couples to get divorced in their fifties, the fastest-growing cohort for separating.

Spirituality: Not a dirty word – our skins get thinner, we are closer to the divine at this point. Existential questions arise that we might not have considered before, like what comes next, or why are we here? What does it all mean? What really matters becomes more pertinent. It is okay to start exploring things you might once have dismissed, to find yourself feeling things rather than rationalising them, to be in truly uncharted territory.

Synchronicity: Noticing signs and symbols that come together to show you you're on the right path – could be as simple as becoming cognisant of and moved by birdsong at sunset, or a bunch of coincidences, or something you need suddenly landing in your life, or a new person arriving for you just when you needed them.

Vanaprastha: A twenty-five-year phase between the ages of fifty and seventy-four. It is part of four Hindu cycles of life – student, householder, hermit/forest dweller, wandering ascetic/holy man – and literally means 'retiring to the forest'. It is the stage when one passes the responsibilities of running a household over to the next generation. One goes from being a householder and being engaged in family life to a more introspective and meditative stage of life. Initially, one will act as a wise elder, providing advice and guidance to those in need. As time passes he/she will gradually withdraw from the world to live a more spiritual and solitary life, going into nature to discover wisdom. The transition to Vanaprastha marks a profound shift in the goals of a person, from being focused on the material pursuits of wealth and pleasure to looking inward, self-realisation and ultimately unity with the divine.

Wallowing: *See* Less-ing – allowing yourself to feel your feelings. If you are grief-stricken after a major loss you will need a bit of time just to be sad, to wallow, to feel the full impact of what has happened. Remember *We're Going on a Bear Hunt*, the kids' story: Can't go over it, can't go under it, got to go through it. There is no shortcut through a big loss. If you don't feel it now and give yourself time, it will bite you on the bum later. Give yourself permission to be finding it tough. Eat chocolate, watch movies, book yourself a holiday. Give yourself some love. *See* Nature *above*, it helps!

ACKNOWLEDGEMENTS

I couldn't have written this book without all of you wonderful Queenagers who have shared your stories and supported my work so generously over the last few years. Thank you to everyone who has become part of Noon, who has come to our retreats and events, sat in our circles, walked up (or slithered down) mountains on our trips, and to all of the amazing women on my Noon Advisory Board who so generously lent their names, reputations and advice to get this project off the ground. Thank you all for saying yes.

Of course, I couldn't have survived this time without the deep love and support of my husband Derek and my daughters Alice and Laura. So much love and gratitude! I love you ALL, always. Also key was Claire Gillis, the 'big sister' who found me in my hour of need and asked: 'What would you do if you weren't afraid?' She then became my co-founder at Noon and the origin of the funds that made it possible. Thank you, Claire. I'd also like to thank my sister Annie Pesskin; my brother Luke Mills, for succour on long walks; Tiffanie Darke, the friend on the bench; Jake Lushington, the brother I chose; Decca Aitkenhead, who took me to Jamaica; my agent Katie Fulford and publisher Lisa Milton; my editor Rachael Kilduff; the brilliant copy-editing of Lorraine Jerram; and all of the team at HarperCollins – after so many years of being an editor myself it has been a *joy* to work with such a skilled and sensitive bunch. Thanks for making this book so much better! And thanks to my namesake and aunt Eleanor

Fein, who so kindly lent me her beautiful house in France when the writing got arduous.

This book is the product of so many conversations with so many Queenagers, particularly: Nancy West, Avivah Wittenberg-Cox, Ayala Gill, Liz Dawes, Tamsin Calidas, Kati Taunt (especially for coming to the women's festival – I'll never forget your face when you emerged from the breathwork!) – and Club 43 (particularly Liz Silk, Jenni Williams, and Widge). Gabby at the pond, Lisa McCauley, Tina Backhouse, Mama Bia and all the Queenagers on the Noon Morocco trip, my Noon team – Jackie Naghten, Jennifer Howze, Karen Stenning, Alison Page, Diane Kenwood, Jocelyn Cripps, Thelma Mensah and Megan Payton. And also Kerensa Jennings, Marianne McDonald, Anoushka Healy, Achara Tait, Kate McMillan, Beatrice Aidin, Eve Pollard, Tree Sherriff, Olivia Lankester, Sarah Belfield, Katie Hickman, Jo Brooks, Sarah Baxter, Margarette Driscoll, Nicci Harrison, Sandra Davis, Sarah Pittendrigh, Liz Mosely, Katie Vanneck-Smith, Justine Roberts, Sheryl Sandberg, Roger Tempest and Paris Ackrill, Rhodri Samuel, Tabitha James Kraan, Dianne Duainn, Minreet, Saeeda, Jarvis, Lesley Thomas, Sally Henzell, Dr Mairi Macleod, Lalita Taylor, Hanneke Smits, June Sarpong, Angie Moxham, Sophie Neary, Helena Morrissey, Danni Hewson, Diana Dugdale, Victoria Whitford, Kirsteen Tait, Julie Owen Moylan, Rachel Peru, Molly Cochrane, Sue Peart, Clare Dubois, Vicky Harper (who ran my first ever Queenager piece and my first article about being whacked in the *Telegraph*), Lindsey Simpson, Kate Muir, Carolyn Harris MP, Jackie Anniesley, Sheila Verajska, Guru Eric, Johann Hari (for all the good advice), Denise, Hannah Tchecho and so many others!

Finally, thanks to my wider family, my mum, my dad, my stepfather Peter, Max, Theo, Tessa, Jessie, Matthew, Pandora, my aunt Nancy (for having me to stay and for reading my articles religiously) and my big sis cousin Tamzin. To all my gorgeous nieces who never fail to brighten my day: Lola, Saskia, Cheski, Delphi, Skye and May, Ottie,

Hero, Leyla, Leonie and baby CC. I hope this book teaches you to look forward to being Queenagers! Plus my sisters-in-law Bree, Ella, Josie and Asia, and my brothers-in-law Alan and Finn. Our family are our greatest teachers.

I feel such a sense of gratitude and amazement that what felt like a death has ended up being so fruitful and joy-filled. I'd also like to thank all the people who shared their stories which have not ended up in the book. Some of the darker, more controversial material got removed in the editing process, but I am coming back to that.

I am aware reading through this book just how privileged my life has been. I was fortunate indeed to get a front-row seat on the unfolding of history during my years as a journalist and to work with some exceptional people. And I had the best education money could buy – thanks for that, Dad! But I hope that despite my privileged perspective some of this journey resonates and can help create a new map for what the later stages of women's lives can look like. A story is the most powerful thing in the world. I hope this one has the power to create change, in however small a way.

If you would like to be a part of our Queenager Revolution at Noon, come and sign up at www.noon.org.uk.

INDEX

sex and pornography 119–124,
    212
therapy
    eidetic imaging 26–27
    shapeshifting 38–41, 42
Thich Nhat Hanh 24–25
Tolle, Eckhart 24
TreeSisters 193, 196–197
trekking 44–51
truth 17–19, 38, 194

uncertainty, facing 23, 25–26, 28,
    185, 279–280
ungloving 289–290

Vanaprastha 260–261, 302

wallowing 12–13, 302
witches 194–195, 282
Wittenberg-Cox, Avivah 143–146,
    147–148
women
    cultural expectations 35, 38
    sistering 193–198
    visibility of 199–201
work *see also* redundancy
    age and wisdom 91

being the breadwinner 76–77,
    163
competitiveness 198
cultural expectations 35–36
experience not respected
    137–139, 154–155
finding purpose 187–192
flexibility 140, 151
glass ceiling 135–136, 149,
    150–154, 156, 160
job hunting 134
loss of sense of self 36–37, 260,
    264
menopause 159–160, 197,
    229–231
mentoring 157, 170
new challenges and reinvention
    139–140, 168–169, 173–175,
    179–181, 189–190
Queenagers leaving 136–138,
    149, 151, 154–159, 160
Queenagers requirements 157
self-employment 189
younger women opting out 144,
    157

Yeoh, Michelle 144, 299